SO-EJV-678

LELORD KORDEL'S
NATURAL FOLK REMEDIES

Also by Lelord Kordel

COOK RIGHT, LIVE LONGER: The Lelord Kordel Cook-book

SECRETS FOR STAYING SLIM

HOW TO KEEP YOUR YOUTHFUL VITALITY AFTER 40

EAT AND GROW YOUNGER

HEALTH THROUGH NUTRITION

LELORD KORDEL'S

NATURAL FOLK REMEDIES

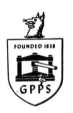

G. P. PUTNAM'S SONS

NEW YORK

Copyright © 1974 by Lelord Kordel

All rights reserved. This book, or parts thereof, must not be reproduced in any form without permission. Published simultaneously in Canada by Longman Canada Limited, Toronto.

SBN: 399-11205-7

Library of Congress Catalog Card Number: 73-78591

PRINTED IN THE UNITED STATES OF AMERICA

Contents

Foreword
Grandma Ate Flowers!

Among my earliest childhood memories are the walks I took with my grandmother through her flower garden. Standing like golden giants against the fence was a long row of sunflowers. At that time, nobody in this country would think of eating sunflowers . . . nobody, that is, except Grandma and me—and the birds!

For somewhere Grandma had read that the Russian and Turkish armies could march all day, with only a pocketful of sunflower seeds to sustain them. So she taught me how to hull the seeds with my teeth and fingers, as the soldiers did.

One day, after lifting me numerous times to reach the tall sunflowers, Grandma picked some lilies of the valley and sat down on the grass to munch them. Always curious, I squatted down beside her and asked, "Are they good, Grandma?"

"Good for a fast heart," she replied. "Is your heart fast?"

"Only when I run. When is yours fast?"

"Only when I lift a heavy boy sky-high a dozen times."

Grandma laughed, tucking the rest of the flowers in her hair. "And tonight, for supper, we're having something even better to slow down a fast heart—asparagus!"

That was my grandmother—a walking encyclopedia of the strangest information. Like the spring day she picked a bachelor button, crushed it and rubbed it on my neck.

"It's time I made an infusion of these," she said, "to keep mosquitoes away and to have on hand as a strengthening tonic."

Infusion . . . strengthening tonic . . . what odd-sounding words to a boy just learning to read. In the months and years that followed, I was also to discover the exotic names of plants that grew in Grandma's garden but rarely appeared in picture books—like comfrey and coltsfoot, horehound and hops, chamomile and mullein, filáree and nettle.

But it was Grandma's vast storehouse of facts that never ceased to amaze me . . . and still does.

Though I was only five years old, can I ever forget that day she sat on the back steps, her straight frame slumped a little, eating honeysuckle? When Grandma saw me peeking through the screen door, she patted the steps in an invitation to join her. With only a faint smile of welcome, she handed me some honeysuckle from the trellised vines around the porch. I was biting the ends off the flowers, sucking the drops of nectar and throwing the rest away, when I noticed that Grandma was eating the whole blossom.

"Nothing like honeysuckle blooms," she said, "to lift the spirits when you're feeling spleenish and downcast." (Two more new words!)

Grandma was always eager to convey her knowledge to others. "Spring crocus," she once told me, "was known as the 'bicarbonate of soda' of medieval times, before folks replaced it with more trustworthy flowers. I never did put much trust in a crocus."

I never did get to ask what she meant by "more trustworthy" flowers, and why she didn't "trust" a crocus! For Grandma had boundless faith in the healing power of nature—a faith she imparted to all around her. But it wasn't faith alone that made her an "authority."

When she and my grandfather were first married, Grandma made home remedies of the same natural substances that her mother and grandmother had used. Before long, she began searching, experimenting, trying out a new remedy or adding extra ingredients to old ones.

Grandma read everything she could get her hands on, from the almanac to Grandpa's chemistry books, an assortment of herbals, and all the medical and scientific books and journals she could borrow from doctors, whom she had no faith in professionally, but who were friends of long standing.

As her family grew, so did her "experiments." Sometimes both got a little out of hand. When that happened, Grandpa would remonstrate, "Why can't you be like other women and leave well-enough alone?"

"Because well-enough isn't good enough," she would answer, "and I want to make it better!"

How could Grandpa fight such "logic"? Secretly, I think, he loved those arguments.

Like the day Grandma proudly invited us all to dinner, to savor her first flower recipes: unopened buds of day lilies dipped in beaten eggs and sautéed, green buds of sunflowers steamed and lightly buttered, a salad consisting of dandelion leaves and blossoms and the leaves and flowers of violets, nasturtiums, and borage.

"How in blazes do you know that these conglomerations won't poison us?" Grandpa growled.

"Because I've already tried them," Grandma said gaily.

And she had. But make no mistake about it: Before testing them herself, Grandma spent many months studying every scrap of information she could lay her hands on.

"Don't you ever go popping flowers or anything else in your mouth unless you know what you're eating," she once warned me sternly. "Some flowers and weeds are good for you, and some can make you sick—even kill you. Until you learn the difference, you be sure to ask me."

In addition to her vast knowledge, my grandmother had a great flair for the dramatic.

"Ralphie Kurnick!" she once shouted at a friend who'd come to play with me. "You go straight home so your mamma can doctor that cold!"

Sniffling sadly, Ralphie peered at me dejectedly through swollen, watery eyes, and started for the door.

"Wait a minute," said Grandma, her face lighting up impishly. "What's Mother doing for that cold?"

Ralphie rubbed his nose on his sleeve and mumbled, "Some pills and stuff."

"Pills! Come back here, Ralphie! You can stay a while if you and Lee play in the garden."

Soon Grandma joined us, carrying honey-sweetened lemonade, rose-hip jelly sandwiches (on homemade bread), and a basket of fresh violets.

As we ate our sandwiches, Ralphie suddenly gawked and sputtered, "Your grandma's eating flowers, leaves and all!"

"Sure," I said matter-of-factly, "flowers taste good. May we have some, Grandma?"

Little did I realize that we'd played right into her hands. After giving us each a handful of violet blossoms and leaves, Grandma vanished into the kitchen.

As Ralphie downed his flower-snack—timidly at first, then with gusto—Grandma returned with a small bundle for him. How strange she must have sounded to the neighbors when she sent Ralphie home, shouting: "Now don't you forget, Ralphie! Tell your mother to give you the honey and horehound night and morning, and two garlic cloves, a spoonful of rose hips, and a fistful of violets every three hours!"

What a performance!

Needless to say, there were lots of people who scoffed at my grandmother, pitied her, laughed behind her back. Some of my friends, with an honesty that is the province of children and saints, even told me that their parents considered Grandma "tetched."

It never troubled me. They were all jealous, I concluded, because even at that early age, I realized that my grandmother was different.

She looked younger, prettier, healthier, and was more fun than other grandmothers. In an emergency or during an illness, she was always the one who knew what to do, promptly and decisively.

It was old, argumentative Grandpa who long ago advised, "Pay attention to your grandma and listen to what she tells you. Someday you'll realize that she's a woman far ahead of her time."

I recalled those words, one day, when a visitor asked Grandma, "Why do you trouble yourself with plants and home remedies when the drugstore carries plenty of patent medicine?"

"Patent fiddlesticks!" Grandma exploded.

I tugged at her apron and promised, "Don't worry about me, Grandma. I'll never take any patent fiddlesticks!"

A smile chased the indignation from her face, and she patted my head. "That's a good boy, Lee. You see that you don't."

More than sixty years have passed, and I still haven't broken that promise. Why should I? My grandmother remained hale and hearty until the day she died . . . at the age of one hundred and one!

Now let's see how science explains it. . . .

1

The Healing Power of Nature's Remedies

When the world was young and unpolluted, nature was the only doctor known to man. Her plants, herbs, roots, and leaves were both food and medicine. Unlike my grandmother, man was *forced* to experiment with them, step by step, slowly learning of their value and how to use them.

As centuries passed, there were doctors to treat him, but those first doctors of record, like early man, had no medicines except the ones extracted from natural sources. There were no drug manufacturers, no chemists—only the chemistry of nature to rely on.

"Let your food be your medicine," wrote Hippocrates, the Father of Medicine. For those who followed him, he left a list of four hundred herbs that were used medicinally in the fourth century B.C. A number of them are still in use in many parts of the world.

Another Greek, Dioscorides, the personal physician of Antony and Cleopatra, compiled a list of six hundred plants and herbs that formed the basis of therapy for several hundred years.

By the fifteenth century, there were numerous books on herbal therapy in Italian, German, and Latin. But the first really comprehensive herbal was published in 1597. It was written by Dr. John Gerard, a British surgeon who was apothecary to King James I. As a physician, surgeon, and herbalist who grew more than one thousand species in his own garden (would Grandma have loved to meet him!), he was well qualified to write the most complete herbal of his time.

The most extensive research, by far, was performed by Nicholas Culpeper, a seventeenth century herbalist. One of his works, *The Compleat Herbal,* is still widely studied by naturopaths and herbalists for its historical value. A passionate advocate of plant therapy, Culpeper ran into frequent conflict with the College of Physicians (a counterpart of today's AMA) whom he dubbed "a proud, insulting, domineering and narrow-minded lot."

In some areas, Nicholas Culpeper made a few exaggerated claims in his prescribing a remedy for nearly every disease imaginable. But, in the process, he succeeded in classifying nearly all the known herbs with thorough descriptions of their medicinal properties. His pioneering groundwork laid the foundation for subsequent theories, remedies, and cures that emerged when research techniques became more sophisticated.

Even today, the writings of Culpeper, and herbalists who followed him, reveal small goblets of scientific information that justify a reappraisal of plants and their medicinal value. But in the razzle-dazzle of mass-produced "wonder" drugs, "up" and "down" pills, synthetic hormones, and capsulized food substitutes, herbal medicine fell into a state of dormancy for several generations.

After all, why waste time mixing Grandma's violet and rosehip concoctions for colds, when all you need is one or two antihistamines a day? Why bother with *any* "home-grown" remedies when there's a plethora of pills for anything that ails you?

One answer comes from Dr. Jeremiah Stamler, head of the Chicago Board of Health's Heart Disease Control Program. Speaking of preventive measures for potential coronary victims, he declared, *"Methods of prevention must be safe, and no one is sure of the long-term effect of drugs. Prevention cannot be based on drugs. If the coronary disease is a product of a way of life of which diet is a factor, then use of drugs is irrational. Diet is better than drugs."* (My italics)

Another voice of caution comes from Britain's Dr. Harry Lilly, who has said, "Drugs patch up the symptoms, not the causes . . . The medical profession on both sides of the Atlantic is being dictated to by the pharmaceutical houses."

Dr. Dale G. Friend, professor of medicine at Harvard and head of Peter Bent Brigham Hospital in Boston, put it most succinctly when he stated, "There is no such thing as a safe drug."

Perhaps that is why, today, we are witnessing a tremendous revival in herbal and folk remedies, natural foods and beauty products. Born of rebellion and disillusionment with the status quo, a generation of young seekers and questioners are going back to nature to find a new way of life. Dissatisfied with the present, out of step with their parents, they are turning to the past in a search for values of proven worth, which can be adapted to their life-styles. In short, the pendulum of public interest has begun to swing full-circle.

Many of the facts have long been evident, and extensive studies are now in progress. A few examples of herbs, plants, and folk remedies that have already proved valuable in modern medicine include:

Rauwolfia, an extract of the snakeroot plant native to India. Used for centuries in the Far East for its calming effect, Rauwolfia is now employed as a tranquilizer in the treatment of mental and emotional disturbances, to lower the blood pressure, and to relieve withdrawal symptoms of narcotics addicts. *Reserpine,* a derivative of rauwolfia, is sold under a number of trade names.

Quinine, derived from the bark of the cinchona tree. Old-time herbalists brewed the bark into a tea to treat "the ague," better known today as the chills and fever of malaria.

Digitalis, obtained from the leaves of the foxglove and other plants. Prescribed today by doctors, as a stimulant to treat disorders of the heart and circulatory system, digitalis was first used in England as a brew. An old Shropshire woman is credited with making the first brew, more than one hundred years ago.

Penicillin, a powerful antibiotic obtained from fungi growing as green mold on such foods as decaying fruit, cheese, and stale bread. Long before penicillin was "discovered," our great-grandmothers were making poultices of moldy bread to cure infections —without the dangerous side effects that some persons get from penicillin.

Ephedrine, from the Chinese plant Ma-huang (a variety of stubby horsetail). It is used in the treatment of bronchial asthma, hay fever, nasal congestion, and to dilate the pupils in eye examinations.

Curare, extracted from a plant of South American origin, now an invaluable aid during surgery. Given in carefully controlled dosages, it relaxes the muscles of the patient undergoing an operation. It is also used to relieve muscle spasms in tetanus and other related conditions.

Rutin, found in buckwheat and rye and in the flowers, rue, hydrangea, and forsythia. It is used to strengthen fragile capillaries and reduce the incidence of recurring hemorrhage in diabetic retinitis and certain forms of pulmonary hemorrhage.

Horehound, licorice root, lemon, honey, and slippery elm were used in various combinations by our forefathers (and my grandmother) to treat coughs, colds and sore throats. Today, you'll find one or more of them in most of the throat lozenges and cough syrups on the market.

These are only a few of the accepted medicines derived from herbs, plants, and other natural sources. Modern scientists are beginning to recognize the debt they owe to nature's healing remedies, and many of these scientists are becoming alarmed over the indiscriminate use of drugs, whether taken by the self-medicator or prescribed by a doctor.

Herbs never cure one disease by creating another, as drugs sometimes do. Herbal and natural remedies work more slowly than drugs, but their action is safe and gentle, and no risk is involved in their long-range use. The continuous use of drugs can and often does produce harmful side effects. In many instances, even those considered safe have proven fatal under certain conditions or in combination with other drugs.

Most of you have heard or read of the tragic, drug-induced deaths of Marilyn Monroe, Dorothy Dandridge, Janis Joplin, Alan Ladd, and columnist Dorothy Kilgallen. Have you any idea what drugs or combination of them might be fatal for *you?*

The doctors themselves are not always sure. They are busy men who are subjected to such a constant barrage of new products from drug and pharmaceutical manufacturers that they have neither the time to absorb the data concerning them nor a way to test their efficacy or potential danger except upon their patients.

Yet, says Dr. Wendell Macleod, dean of medicine at the University of Saskatchewan, Canada, "Confidence in the healing power of nature has been displaced by undue dependence upon the popular drugs of the moment." Dr. Macleod urges us to "get back to nature" and renew our faith in her healing power.

Perhaps his message has been heard, for here in America the

movement has already begun. Until recently the search for natural and herbal remedies and other products was mainly a project of the young back-to-nature groups and the concerned health-seekers of all ages. But now help is coming from unexpected sources, including a branch of the United States government.

A search, currently under way in parts of Texas and Mexico to find and classify medicinal plants used in folk medicine, is being made on a grant from the National Institute of Mental Health of HEW's Health Services and Mental Health Administration.

Compared with other government grants, this one is very small, but the fact that the government is sponsoring a study of herbal remedies at all is a sign of changing attitudes. And Women's Lib should be pleased that the project is headed by a woman, Dr. Clarissa T. Kimber, of Texas A & M Foundation at College Station, Texas.

Dr. Kimber's search will be for both the cultivated and wild medicinal plants that are believed to be among the first used in medicine in this country. Some of them are in danger of becoming extinct, unless the sources of the wild varieties that are dying out can be found and placed under cultivation. When found, those with medicinal properties that can be utilized will be sent to researchers for further chemical study.

In the meantime, another search for safe, natural substances has been going on at the Mayo Clinic. Their researchers have found one substance in yellow clover which may replace heparin and dicoumarin for dissolving blood clots without producing undesirable side effects.

A progressive new program was developed recently by Dr. John R. Hogness, president of the Institute of Medicine, for American doctors to go to China to study Chinese medical techniques, including herbal therapy. And Dr. Samuel Rosen, recently returned from China and a study of their age-old therapy, is quoted by the New York *Times* as saying, "I have seen the past, and it works."

Their heritage of the past and scientific knowledge of the present combine to give the Russian people their amazing health and vitality. According to a statement describing the collaboration of Soviet scientists and the Medical Academy, herbal remedies constitute 40 percent of Russia's curative therapy. In the Soviet Union there are now more than one thousand herbs that are used medicinally.

The Bible tells us, "The fruit of the tree is for man's meat, and the leaves for his medicine" (Ezekiel 47:12).

Make the leafy greens and other healthful, edible herbs part of your diet as often as possible—as my grandmother did—and learn which ones have specific therapeutic value in certain conditions. Best of all, plan to "let your food be your medicine" by including a variety of herbs in each week's menu as salad greens, vegetables, and herb teas.

By consistently using herbs and plants to build better health and to strengthen your body's resistance to disease, you will find yourself resorting less and less to dangerous drugs. And before long you, too, will join the swelling ranks of ex-skeptics who have rediscovered the healing power of nature's "pharmaceutical factory."

2

The Real Flower Power

After some fifty years as a writer, lecturer, and consultant in my field, I'm still considered by many to be a bit of an eccentric, that is to say, a professional "nutrition nut." Consequently I'm subjected to a constant cascade of criticism, ranging from angry invective to bemused tolerance. And, for some strange reason, the loudest protests come from persons half my age, who look—and feel—twice as old!

All my disputants share one common belief—that we "food faddists" are *suffering*. Sure, they concede, proper food habits make for a stronger body, a sounder mind, a sunnier disposition —but is all that worth the "sacrifice" of gourmet eating?

Frankly, I still don't know what it takes to become a full-fledged, certified, nose-in-the-air gourmet, but if my friend Harry Stevens is any example, gourmets are always great for a few laughs. Harry, a member of every culinary club within a hundred-mile radius, was positively chagrined the first time he came to dinner at the Kordels'.

"Lelord!" he gasped, nearly choking on his cocktail onion. "Don't you ever let up?"

I knew what was coming and decided to play it cool. "Let up on what, Harry?"

"That leaf you're crushing. I mean, considering how little you imbibe, do you have to pollute your highballs with that stuff, too?"

"This 'stuff'," I said, emptying the powdered leaf into my

glass, "helps to calm the nerves, prevent insomnia, and strengthen the heart muscles."

"Uh-oh"—Harry laughed—"I hear your grandmother talking again."

"Guess again, Harry. Grandma never touched hard liquor. I was introduced to this concoction in a London pub."

"You're kidding!" A familiar look of skepticism crept over his face. "Since when have the British been spiking their booze with medicine?"

"Tell me, Harry, do you object to mint leaves in a julep?"

"Well—no, I guess not."

"How about lemon peels in martinis, cinnamon bark in hot rum, buffalo grass in vodka?"

"Enough! I surrender!" Cautiously, Harry approached the dish of leaves on the serving tray. "What's this stuff called?"

"Borage," I said.

"Borage," he repeated, wincing. "It even *sounds* like a medicine."

"Would you care to sample some, Harry? One thing I guarantee—it won't kill you."

Gingerly, he brought the dish to his wrinkled nose and sniffed. "Not bad," he said, the wrinkle suddenly vanishing. He picked up a leaf, scrutinized it for a long moment, then popped it into his mouth.

"Hey!" he exclaimed delightedly. "If I didn't know better, I'd say it was cucumber! And I love cucumbers!"

"So do the English," I said. "That's why so many of them add borage to their highballs—for flavor and coolness. They also savor the chopped leaves and flowers raw, in salads, or steamed, seasoned with butter and lemon juice."

"Okay, Lelord"—Harry sighed—"I'm hooked. Tell me more."

I told Harry that the borage plant, with its exquisite blue star-shaped flowers, has been used to treat a variety of ailments since the early days of the Greeks. A widely quoted Greek proverb says, "I, Borage, always bring courage." The Welsh name for borage means "herb of gladness." Dioscorides called it "a nerve tonic of rare virtue," and recommended it to relieve depressed moods and numerous other ailments.

"Hold it!" Harry interrupted. "This Dioscorides, whoever he was. Just because he says so, why do I have to take his word for it?"

"You don't," I replied. "But even the most skeptical modern researchers have found valid reasons for some of his claims. Take *their* word for it."

An analysis of the plant, I explained, has shown it to be a good source of calcium and potassium, the organic minerals so vital in calming nerves, controlling tensions, preventing insomnia, and, in general, keeping one from becoming a nervous wreck. They're also valuable in relaxing and strengthening the heart and other muscles, which probably accounts for borage's reputation as a heart tonic.

"Is it any wonder," I added, "that a plant containing two such beneficial minerals has a centuries-old reputation, in all parts of the world, as a remedy for many different conditions?"

In France a hot tea made of dried or fresh borage flowers and leaves is used as a soothing treatment for feverish colds. Taken two or three times a day and before retiring, borage's cooling properties help reduce the fever, soothe the bronchials and digestive system, and make the patient generally more comfortable.

In Arabia it was once the custom to eat borage leaves and flowers raw, as a mild stimulant and "to strengthen the heart and limbs." I don't know whether modern Arabs have outgrown that custom or not. If they have, it would be a good idea for them (and for all of us) to revive it.

That's because modern research has found that borage leaves are beneficial in stimulating the adrenal glands. When those vital glands are nudged into action, it does indeed have the effect of "strengthening the heart and limbs." For adrenalin, released into the bloodstream, is capable of producing superhuman strength and courage to meet disaster or an unexpected emergency. This is what the Greeks really meant when they declared, "I, Borage, always bring courage."

In Arabia, too, many generations of mothers have consumed borage leaves and flowers to increase their milk while nursing. As many young mothers of today are beginning to recognize the advantages of breast-feeding, that's another old custom well worth reviving.

British herbalists recommend borage tea to keep the kidneys and bladder healthy and to prevent the disorders common to those organs. As a natural, effective diuretic, borage is widely used throughout Europe. The English have also found it to be an effective blood purifier, nerve tonic, and mild stimulant.

"Fine, Lelord," Harry said, "you've convinced me about borage. But I noticed, growing in your garden, a bed of catnip. Are you going to tell me . . ."

"That I eat catnip, too?" I broke in. "Absolutely. Or rather, I drink it—frequently."

"What does it do? Turn you on? Like a cat?"

"No, Harry, 'turning on' is strictly for potheads and junkies. And I suppose cats *are* 'junkies' when it comes to catnip. But on humans it has an entirely different effect."

"Like what?" he drawled suspiciously.

For years, I told Harry, catnip has been listed in numerous pharmacopoeias as a nervine, mild stimulant, tonic and anti-spasmodic. It has also been proven effective against gastric distress and fever.

"So has bicarbonate of soda, which is a lot easier to come by." Harry laughed.

"True," I said. "So are most patent medicines. I'd never deny that."

"So why bother with catnip?"

"Because it's safer and a lot healthier."

Laboratory analyses of catnip, I went on, have shown it to be a good source of vitamins A and C, and probably a number of other vitamins and minerals.

The Pennsylvania Dutch seem to be most aware of the benefits of catnip as a tea. They give it to babies and children, sometimes sweetened with a little honey and diluted with milk. Adults drink a cup of hot catnip tea after meals, as an aid to digestion, and at bedtime, as a relaxing nightcap to induce sleep. Some of the robust old-timers claim that there's no finer tonic than a cup of hot or cold catnip tea before each meal.

But the Pennsylvania Dutch are not alone. Generations of mothers, all over the world, feed two or three teaspoons of the warm tea to relieve their infants of the colic. Babies find it very soothing.

"Great," Harry said, "but how does it taste?"

"Harry," I answered, reaching into a jar of dried leaves, let's get one thing straight. I never eat anything that tastes bad unless my doctor orders it."

As he started to reply, I popped a leaf into his mouth. "Catnip?" he sputtered, bewildered.

I nodded, watching his amazement grow.

"It tastes like mint," he said.

"Why shouldn't it?" I said. "Catnip is a member of the mint family. The same family that includes peppermint and spearmint."

"Okay, I'll buy that, Lelord. Borage for courage, catnip for colic. But what about a guy like me, who suffers from ulcers? Have you got a cure for that?"

"Harry," I chided, "the way you gorge yourself at those gourmet gatherings, nothing can cure your ulcers. But if you're looking to relieve the pain, try red clover."

"R-red c-clover," he stammered. "All of a sudden, milk isn't good enough."

"I never said that. Milk is fine, but it doesn't have the demulcent properties of red clover. The next time your ulcers act up, try combining your milk with red clover tea, preferably between meals. You may find it relieving a few other symptoms, too."

"Such as . . . ?"

I told Harry that red clover tea is good for many types of stomach distress, including mild indigestion and excess acidity. "But most of all," I said, "modern herbalists prize red clover blossoms as a good source of calcium and phosphorus."

For many years, scientists have known that children suffering from rickets, the terrible disease that turns them bowlegged, lack phosphorus in their diets. Hand in hand with rickets goes defective teeth. Even I chuckled at my grandmother when she urged me to eat red clover blossoms for my bones and teeth—until I learned that phosphorus acts as a hardening agent that helps strengthen the bones and teeth.

Other symptoms of phosphorus deficiency are loss of appetite, loss of weight, general weakness, and "feeling-bad-all-over" symptoms. Long before it was known as a source of essential minerals, red clover was used successfully as a tonic to overcome those conditions. A small cupful of red clover tea, before each meal and at bedtime, often works wonders.

Among others who benefit from red clover's soothing demulcent action are sufferers from spasmodic asthma, coughs, and bronchitis. Mothers have found it helpful in easing the strain of severe attacks in children with whooping cough.

"All this sounds great, Lelord," said Harry, "but with all these teas you're recommending, I'd wind up *floating* to bed every night. Aren't there other ways to enjoy a flower-food?"

"You might try one of my favorite snacks," I said. "White clover honey."

"*White* clover honey. Is white clover any different from red clover?"

"In many ways they're similar, though the effects of white clover are a lot less powerful. By the way, Harry, have your kids had the mumps yet?"

"Just my oldest boy. The other two are still candidates."

"Well," I said, "try this for size . . ."

And I told Harry of white clover's one unique talent that no other flower seems to possess: its effectiveness in warding off mumps. In many parts of England, when a mumps epidemic threatens a community, people who aren't already immune drink white clover tea as a preventive. If no dried clover tea is available, and the blossoms are out of season, they eat the honey as a substitute.

"Either way, Harry, you can't go wrong with white clover. Both the tea and honey are healthy *and* delicious."

Harry chuckled, "I'm beginning to suspect that you consider *all* flowers delicious."

"Harry," I said, "it may shock you to learn that we 'nature freaks' have the same taste buds as you 'normal' eaters. Some foods I love, some I don't care for, no matter how healthful. With flowers, as with any other delicacy, I have my favorites."

"Fair enough. Now suppose I just couldn't stand the taste of, say, catnip. Should I *force* myself to eat it?"

"Not at all. Even I'd get tired of a flower if I had to eat it every day. There's enough variety in the plant kingdom to satisfy every palate. The dandelion, for instance, contains some of the same wholesome elements as borage, catnip, and clover."

That was no cop-out. Dandelion leaves, rich in vitamin C, have long been known as a preventive and remedy for scurvy. They contain more vitamin A than other leafy greens (except violet leaves) and are a good source of calcium and potassium. In addition, they're loaded with more iron than spinach.

The curative powers of dandelion act on the stomach, liver, kidneys, and bladder, often with amazing speed. The entire plant contains natural nutritive salts that act as a blood cleanser and tonic, and reduce the acid content of the blood.

The green leaves, eaten raw in salads, lightly steamed as a vegetable, or made into a tea, are effective as a diuretic and remedy for edema (dropsy), an aid to increasing the activity of the liver and stomach, and a stimulant to the spleen. Because of its stimulating effect on the pancreas, improvement has been noted in diabetics who include dandelion greens and/or tea in their diet several times a week.

"Scurvy! Edema! Diabetes!" Harry snorted. "Fat chance I have of contracting one of those illnesses!"

"Statistically speaking, you're right," I said. "That's why I wouldn't urge you to make dandelions—or any other plant, for that matter—a *must* in your diet. I merely recommend them as tasty, harmless *preventives*. For the more common, everyday complaints, there are many others to choose from."

"Like what?"

"Your wife, for example, might go for a tea brewed from the flowers of the feverfew, a popular eighteenth-century remedy for so-called ladies' ailments."

"Is that why feverfew is also called bachelor's buttons?" Harry quipped. "Those eighteenth-century chicks had a great sense of humor."

"So do you, Harry, but I think it was called bachelor's buttons because, as a relief from nervous tension and headaches, it worked just as well on bachelors—and married men, too."

"What else would you recommend for the everyday brand of ailments?"

I told Harry about hollyhock, whose leaves and flowers possess valuable soothing properties that help relieve inflamed mucous membranes in all parts of the body. A tea made of the flowers soothes the digestive tract and has a healing influence on sore mouths and irritated throats. Its soothing quality makes it useful in treating coughs and chest complaints. Among Arab women hollyhock is used as a treatment for inflammation of the uterus and vagina.

Then, of course, I had to mention honeysuckle, my grandmother's favorite remedy for what she called "feeling spleenish." To chase her blues away, Grandma would eat a small handful of fresh blossoms and a few leaves twice a day. If Harry weren't starting to quake like a hypochondriac, I'd have also stressed honeysuckle's beneficial effects on asthma and other respiratory disorders, on rheumatism and general stiffness of the joints.

I did tell him that gypsies consider honeysuckle, mixed with honey and half-dark molasses, a remedy for practically all skin disorders. They also find it to be a gentle, natural laxative.

"Whether or not the gypsies are exaggerating," I added, "you can't go wrong with their tasty blend. Rich in iron, it also provides considerable calcium and some of the B-vitamins. Perhaps that's why honeysuckle is reported to benefit the heart, decrease retention of fluid in the tissues, and reduce the swelling of glands."

"There you go again," Harry said, "making me worry about every ache and pain in my system."

"Sorry about that, Harry. The trouble with us 'health buffs' is, we sometimes get carried away. Let me change the subject a little by recommending an excellent breath-freshener."

"That's better, What's it called?"

"Lavender."

"You mean the same stuff that goes into all those great-smelling perfumes and after-shave lotions?"

"Right. But while your perfumes contain poisonous chemical additives that limit them to 'external use only,' a pure, thick brew of lavender flowers and top shoots makes a great mouthwash. When used regularly, it has a strengthening effect on the gums. Personally, I find that it leaves my mouth feeling clean and refreshed."

British herbalists have found that lavender is also highly nervine. "The next time you have a nervous stomach or sick headache," I advised Harry, "try a cup of hot lavender tea made of fresh or dried flowers. Because the flowers are so strongly scented, you might find the flavor too strong for your taste. In that case, you might enjoy it more by mixing a few blossoms with any other herb tea of your choice."

"Thanks for the tip," Harry said, "but to tell you the truth, when I get a headache, it's not just a headache. It's a *headache!* You know what I mean? It keeps me awake half the night. Pretty soon, from all the tossing and turning, even my joints start to ache."

"What you need," I said, "is a cup of hot primrose tea at bedtime."

That's because the magnesium in primroses makes the tea a soothing drink that helps reduce tension and nervousness. Add milk to it, and you get the additional nerve-relaxing benefits of calcium.

"You know, Lelord, there's one trouble with all these flower remedies," Harry said. "I'm a busy man, and my wife works, too. I haven't got the time to raise a garden."

"Most flower remedies," I said, "are available in health food stores—in their dried form. But there's at least one flower that you can get fresh, in practically any supermarket."

"There is? Which one?"

"The pumpkin."

"Pumpkins! Great! I love pumpkin pie and pudding."

"Did it ever occur to you that you're wasting the best part of the pumpkin when you throw away the flowers, fruit, and seeds?"

"How come?"

I gave Harry another tea recipe: three pumpkin blossoms to a half-pint of boiling water. For generations, this brew has served as a tonic and general builder-upper.

The fruit (or vegetable) of pumpkin—baked, steamed, or raw, finely grated—is also a tonic food, high in nutritive values and strengthening properties, easily digested and soothing to delicate stomachs. Medical experts agree that raw pumpkin is far superior to cooked.

Since ancient times the seeds of the pumpkin have been known as a preventive and remedy for worm infestation, including tapeworm. More recent research indicates that pumpkin seeds contain elements that have been called the building stones for the male hormones. Many doctors recommend the seeds as an aid in maintaining the health of the prostate gland.

"Now we're on the same wavelength!" Harry said eagerly, jotting a note in his memo book. "What other flower-food can I get in the local stores?"

"The sunflower plant," I said, "isn't sold anywhere except in flower shops. But shelled, ready-to-eat sunflower *seeds* are available in all health food stores—and it's the seeds that contain most of the sunflower's healing and nutritive power."

For centuries, I explained, herbalists valued sunflowers for their antimalarial, diuretic, and expectorant properties. Loaded with proteins, minerals, and vitamins, sunflower seeds contain generous amounts of the substances useful in lowering blood cholesterol and preventing the fatty deposits that block arteries and damage the heart.

A study made by American and British dentists, in countries where sunflower seeds are eaten regularly, has shown that people have remarkably healthy gums and strong, sound teeth. That's because these seeds have a high content of phosphorus, calcium in easily assimilated form, and a trace of fluorine—all of which promote dental health and slow down tooth decay. In addition, all that chewing provides the stimulation and exercise that make spongy, bleeding gums firm and healthy, often in a relatively short time.

Being rich in vitamins A and B-2, plus other nutrients, sunflower seeds are of value in correcting night blindness. They also strengthen eyes that are sensitive to the glare of sunlight.

"Keep going, Lelord!" Harry was flying now. "What else can I buy in a candy store?"

"Nothing else I can think of." I could almost hear the thud of his bulky body dropping back to earth. "And that's too bad, Harry, because a lot of people are missing out on one of the most important of all vitamins—the vitamin that Dr. Linus Pauling and other researchers have called a virtual cure for colds and flu."

"Sure," Harry said, "I remember reading about it. Vitamin C. How am I missing out on it?"

"By not including rose hips in your diet, the way the Greeks did, a thousand years before Christ."

And that was no exaggeration. The ancient Greeks prepared rose petals and rose hips in such delectable ways that they were called food for the gods. It took science many more centuries to discover the enormous quantity of vitamin C contained in the hips—the swellings at the base of the flower that enclose the seeds.

Another fine source of vitamin C that goes back to ancient times are violets. Though not nearly so laden with vitamin C as rose hips, violets also contain a high quality of vitamin A, higher than any other leafy greens.

"To add color and flavor to your meals as you boost your vitamin intake," I said to Harry, "try adding the blossoms and chopped leaves to salads, or use them as a garnish."

"Are you *sure* it'll work for me?" he asked.

"Let me put it this way, Harry. As a boy, I ate the blossoms by the handful, and I have never had a cold in my life. Does that make it worth a try?"

"I guess it does. Now may we start eating?"

Poor Harry. I not only bent his ear, I also gave him hunger pangs. I could have gone on and on, but no matter how I garnished my praise of flowers, it all would have added up to one basic fact:

Whether you make them into a syrup, drink them as a tea, nibble them raw, eat them in a salad, cook the leaves with other greens, or make them into internal and external remedies, flowers are, as one ancient herbalist put it, "healing, helpful, and in no way hurtful."

FLOWER RECIPES FROM
AROUND THE WORLD

**Aids to
Digestion**

Dandelion Tea

From England: British herbalists recommend an infusion of dandelion leaves and flowers for chronic disorders of the digestive organs, liver, and kidneys.

Take four ounces of the tea, either hot or cold, three times a day.

From Holland: Dandelion in its various forms is an accepted remedy as a general aid to health. Also as an iron-rich tonic for the anemic.

Primrose Blossoms

A small handful of raw, shredded primrose blossoms and three or four chopped leaves added to the daily diet. Eat as a snack food, combined with salad greens, or use as a garnish for other foods.

Gypsies use primrose as a preventive and remedy for such diverse conditions as high blood pressure and gall bladder complaints, as well as acidity.

Violet Tea

An infusion of dried violet tea or fresh violets before meals has a cooling, healing effect on the mucous membranes, and a beneficial influence on stomach inflammation and ulcers.

Honeysuckle for Liver and Spleen

A decoction of ¾ cup of leaves and ¼ cup blossoms simmered in a pint of water.

Take a small cupful twice a day before meals.

Catnip Tea

The tea is prepared by making an infusion. But instead of the usual one teaspoonful of dried herbs to each cup of boiling water, use two of catnip. Let it steep, covered, for five or ten minutes, to reach the desired strength. Sweeten with honey, if you like. Drink plain or with lemon or a little milk, according to taste.

If you're taking catnip tea as a tonic, the lemon is preferred because of its vitamin C content.

To soothe the nerves and stomach and as a relaxing bedtime drink to induce sleep, the calcium in milk helps make it a natural lullaby drink. (Cats love it with milk, and you know how relaxed they are.)

Lavender Tea

A cup of hot lavender tea made of fresh or dried flowers will calm a nervous stomach and ease a sick headache.

If the scent and flavor are too strong for your taste, mix a few blossoms with any other herb tea of your choice.

Asthma and Respiratory Disorders

Honeysuckle

A strong infusion or a decoction of both the blossoms and leaves soothes the mucous membrane and aids in the expulsion of mucus.

Or chop the leaves into shreds, bruise the blossoms, and combine the two with enough honey to hold them together. Eat the raw mixture by the spoonful as often as needed to soothe the mucous membranes and prevent coughing.

A gypsy variation: As above, except that half honey and half dark molasses are used. The addition of dark molasses makes it an iron-rich remedy and provides considerable calcium and some B vitamins.

Gypsies consider it a remedy for practically all skin disorders and praise its merits as a gentle, natural laxative.

Red Clover

To a cup of hot red clover tea add a squeeze of lemon and a tablespoon of honey.

Drink as needed to relieve coughs and congestion and soothe the bronchials.

Breath Sweeteners

Lavender

A decoction of the flowers and top shoots makes a mouthwash that, when used regularly, has a strengthening effect on the gums and tends to promote their health.

After trying it myself, I can recommend it as a breath sweetener that leaves your mouth feeling clean and refreshed.

Cough Remedies

Borage Syrup

> 1 cup borage juice (*see* Nerve Tonics)
> 2 cups honey
> juice of 2 lemons

Bring borage juice and honey to a boil in a saucepan, stirring constantly. Remove from the fire and stir in lemon juice. Pour into a bottle or jar and cap tightly.

Take 1 to 2 tablespoons as needed. For a cough or sore throat, let it trickle slowly down the throat to give the benefit of its soothing, healing effect.

If a hot drink is desired, stir a tablespoonful of borage syrup into a freshly brewed cup of borage tea.

As a natural healthful sweetener, omit the lemon juice and use simple borage syrup to add sweetness, flavor, and coolness to limeade, lemonade, iced tea, etc.

For a nonalcoholic highball, add ice cubes and a slice of lemon or lime to club soda and stir in a jigger of borage syrup. For extra stimulation with no side effects, try two jiggers.

Red Clover Cough Syrup

> 1 pint honey
> 1 pint water
> 1 ounce red clover blossoms

Clover blossoms should be freshly gathered and thoroughly washed. Heat honey and water to boiling. Add clover blossoms. Simmer gently fifteen minutes. Remove from fire, let stand until cool. Refrigerate.

Take one or two tablespoonfuls as often as needed.

Rose Hips Puree

> 2 pounds, washed, drained, rose hips
> 1½ pints water

Use stainless steel or enamel saucepan. Put rose hips into boiling water; cover and bring to a boil again. Simmer gently until very tender, about fifteen to twenty minutes. (Overcooking causes a loss of flavor and vitamin content.) Press through a fine sieve or put in a blender at low speed until pureed to a jellylike consistency.

Take one or two tablespoons at bedtime and as needed during the day to soothe irritated bronchials and prevent coughing.

Sweeten with honey, thin it with fruit juice, and you have a delicious sauce for dessert.

Rose Hips Sauce

½ cup rose hips puree
½ cup orange or pineapple juice
3 tablespoons honey (or to taste)
2 teaspoons lemon juice

Bring puree, juice, and honey to a boil. Add lemon juice. Take one or two tablespoons at bedtime and as needed during the day to soothe irritated bronchials and prevent coughing. Use as a topping for custard, puddings, gelatin, and ice cream.

Sunflower Cordial

½ cup sunflower seeds
1 quart cold water
grated peel of one lemon
¾ cup honey
2 cups double-strength comfrey tea

Combine sunflower seeds and water in a saucepan and simmer slowly until the liquid is reduced to about a pint. Remove from the fire, strain, stir in the lemon peel, honey, and comfrey tea (available in health-food stores).

Two tablespoonfuls as often as needed to relieve coughing and soothe bronchials.

From Russia: A decoction similar to the above, but with ½ cup of sunflower leaves added, is used not only for pulmonary ailments but for nervous disorders.

Violet Syrup

½ pound fresh violets and stems
2 cups water
1 cup honey
¼ cup almond oil

Bring water to a boil. Place violets in a large glass jar. Add boiling water. Cover and leave to infuse overnight. Strain the blossoms from the liquid, add honey, and return the mixture to the fire. Allow it to come almost, but not quite, to a boil. Add almond oil; mix well. Pour into bottle or jar with tightly fitting cover.

Take as often as needed. If fresh violets are not available, dried violet tea makes an acceptable substitute.

**External
Remedies:
Lotions and
Poultices**

Red Clover Skin Rash Poultice

Make a strong infusion of red clover tea, letting it steep for at least thirty minutes. (Or make a decoction by simmering it gently in boiling water for fifteen to twenty minutes.) Using a piece of absorbent cotton, apply the warm solution to the rash or skin eruption and allow to dry. Repeat as often as necessary, using fresh cotton each time.

For faster results and to prevent a recurrence of the problem, combine the external applications with an internal remedy of tea made of either fresh or dried red clover as a blood-cleansing tonic.

If you have fresh blossoms, try chopping a few of them into salads. Use them as a garnish for cream soups, vegetables, and meats, or add a small amount to any cooked vegetable.

Daisy Lotion and Poultice
Caution: For External Use Only!

A strong infusion or decoction of the leaves can be used as a lotion on wounds, cuts, bruises, and other skin disorders.

To make a poultice, place a pint of leaves in a blender with just enough witch hazel to moisten, reduce to a pulp. Spread on a piece of gauze or a clean cloth and apply to the injury.

The pulped leaves combined with an equal amount of vaseline or pure cold cream, and mixed well, can be used as a healing ointment.

Dandelion Cure for Warts and Corns

Pick a dandelion leaf or flower and squeeze the broken stem until it exudes a drop of milky juice. Apply juice to the wart and allow it to dry. Repeat for two or three consecutive days. The wart will gradually turn dark and fall off, leaving the skin smooth and unblemished. The same treatment is reported to work equally as well for corns. (These remedies are from a gypsy friend.)

Borage Eye Lotion

To refresh tired, burning eyes and help get the red out, use a strong infusion of fresh or dried borage leaves and flowers. Allow to cool slightly, dip pads of cotton into it, and press lightly to remove excess moisture (just enough to prevent dripping). Place pads over eyes for ten or fifteen minutes. If pads become dry, replace them with freshly moistened ones.

Borage Skin Rash Poultice

In a blender, add three tablespoons of water to one cup of carefully washed, fresh chopped borage leaves. Blend to a thick pulp. Spread pulped leaves on a piece of gauze or a clean white cloth and apply to affected area.

Pulped borage leaves make an excellent remedy for hard-to-cure skin rashes, including stubborn and unsightly ringworm.

Honeysuckle Lotion

American Indians boiled honeysuckle leaves in water to make a lotion to promote the healing of wounds and sores.

Honeysuckle lotion is also excellent as a mouthwash and gargle for mouth and throat irritations.

Honeysuckle Poultice

For injuries that require the longer-lasting effects of a poultice, spread the pulped leaves or the pounded roots on a clean cloth or piece of gauze and apply to the wound.

Feverfew Insect Repellant

To repel gnats, mosquitos, and other insects, make a strong infusion of the flowers and leaves. Sponge it on the skin and allow to dry.

I've used it since I was a child and have found that it works better than any mosquito repellant on the market. And feverfew has a pleasant smell!

The pulped leaves and flowers, spread on gauze and applied to the affected parts, have proved useful as a pain-soothing poultice, particularly effective in the treatment of hemorrhoids.

Tonics and Stimulants

Candied Borage Stars

1 egg white, unbeaten
1 tablespoon fresh orange juice
borage flowers
sifted granulated sugar*

Combine egg white and orange juice and beat with a fork until slightly fluffy but not stiff. Use fully opened, carefully washed, borage flowers. Dip flowers in the egg mixture, coating them thoroughly, dipping a second time if necessary. Spread sugar* over them. When they are dry enough not to stick together, place in a covered glass bowl or cookie tin, with waxed paper between each layer of flowers. Refrigerate. May also be frozen for later use.

Rose petals and violets may be candied the same way.

Honeysuckle

Make a decoction from a combination of the leaves and honeysuckle blossoms. Or just eat a small handful of the fresh blossoms and a few leaves twice a day, as grandma did to chase her blues away.

Honeysuckle Bark

A decoction of honeysuckle bark is reported to benefit the heart, decrease retention of fluid in the tissues, and reduce the swelling of glands.

---

* As most of my readers know, I am opposed to the use of white sugar, but this recipe is one of the few exceptions I've made to my rule of avoiding white sugar and products that contain it. In this case the small amount of sugar used isn't enough to offset the healthful properties of the flowers. These dainty confections are meant to be nibbled, not eaten indiscriminately.

Borage Juice

Wash the leaves, shred them with a sharp knife or a pair of kitchen shears, add a little water, place them in a blender set at medium speed. Let mix to a smooth consistency, adding more water if the mixture becomes too thick. (If you use a vegetable juicer instead of a blender you needn't shred the leaves.)

Store the refreshing, mucilaginous juice in jars and use it to add a mineral-rich coolness and flavor to any summer drink of your choice. It freezes well, too, if you want to save a few jars to add to your Christmas and New Year's drinks, and you won't need alcohol to exhilarate you. Remember, the old-time herbalists learned centuries ago that borage "maketh the mind merrie and joyful."

3

Hints on Preparing
Nature's Remedies

As you may have already gathered, some flower remedies are as simple as eating the blossoms or leaves of certain plants. Others require specific preparation, some more and some less.

For remedies that require fresh flowers, growing a few yourself can be a surprisingly easy and pleasant hobby. All it takes is some packages of seed or cuttings, and just a little bit of yard space. If you're an apartment-dweller, you'll be amazed to discover how many different varieties you can raise in one or two window boxes.

But maybe your thumb hasn't the slightest tinge of green, and you've barely enough space to turn around in. If that's the case, your best bet is to make friends with a neighbor who has a flower garden, or find a place where wildflowers grow.

My own yard provides many of the flowers that we use, freshly picked and raw, in salads or make into remedies and recipes. However, because my time is tightly budgeted, I like to keep a supply of the dried varieties on hand for quick preparation.

You might start by buying packaged teas from your local health food store. Some of these stores also carry packets of dried roots and powder. If they are not available there, your pharmacist can order them from his wholesale source.

The dried, packaged herbs, flowers, and teas that you buy at herbalists and in health food stores are organically grown and safe to consume. If you use fresh flowers, be sure they're thoroughly washed and free from the residue of insecticide sprays.

To keep yourself from getting discouraged and bogged down with complicated directions right from the start, it's a good idea to begin with recipes that take a minimum of time and effort. If you like, you can always work up to the tougher ones later.

If you can make a cup of tea, you can make an *infusion,* because that's essentially what it is. Just put the fresh or dried leaves or blossoms—whichever the remedy calls for—in a teapot with freshly boiling water, put the lid on, and let it steep for five to ten minutes, depending on the strength desired. If you brew it too strong, you can always add water after it's strained and ready to drink.

In the absence of a teapot, a glass jar will pinch-hit fine. Just be sure that it has a lid, so you can cover it while the flowers steep.

A *decoction* is similar to an infusion, only stronger. It's made by simmering the plant-parts in boiling water from ten to twenty minutes or until the desired strength is reached.

Roots, stalks, and seeds are usually the parts that require boiling to extract the strength from them. Certain leaves and blossoms, especially tightly closed buds, may also require the stronger method of *decoction.*

For some recipes, the blossoms, leaves, or roots are dried and reduced to a powder. Mixed with the proper liquids, the powder becomes a tonic, cough syrup, or other internal remedy.

Blend the powder with lanolin, Vaseline, or pure cold cream, and you have a healing salve or ointment for external use.

Dissolve it in witch hazel or other specified liquid to make a healing lotion, astringent, or liniment for external application only. Mix it with just enough liquid to form a paste, and you can spread it on a clean piece of cloth for a poultice.

Does it already sound too complicated? Are you tempted to chuck the whole business, race out to the drugstore and load up on aspirin, antihistamine, and all the other ready-to-eat, easy-to-buy, factory-made chemical concoctions?

Or are you still willing to "gamble" the little time and effort it takes to develop a taste for some great new delicacies? You don't have to savor them all: The world of flowers, like the counter in your supermarket, contains a wealth of taste-sensations.

Who knows? If you get to like enough of them, you may never have to touch another patented pill.

4

Kitchen Cures for Whatever Ails You

How often has it happened—in one form or other? You awaken from a good night's sleep, relaxed and refreshed. You're eager to get to the office because a contract will be waiting on your desk, good for a few thousand in commissions. You inhale a lungful of fresh, clean country air and listen to the birds singing in the sunlight. *Wow, what a beautiful day!* You can't wait to get started.

But the oil burner is out of whack, so there's no hot water for your shower. Your wife discovers she's run out of coffee, and, in her agitation, overcooks the eggs. The car has trouble starting, you miss your train, and the train you finally catch is creeping with engine trouble. Arriving at work an hour and a half late, you find not a contract but a telegram canceling the deal!

Oh, what an ugly day! You sink into your chair, trying to collect your confused thoughts, when suddenly it strikes out of nowhere—a wrenching, pounding, buzzing, skull-splitting headache!

Almost everyone who has lived or worked under pressure is familiar with this type of headache. It occurs without other symptoms and is caused by some form of mental stress—in other words, by tension.

Suppressed emotions—like anger, envy, anxiety, fear, and frustration—are common causes of tension headaches. So is racing a deadline to finish a difficult job. When the deadline is met, or if the suppressed emotions can find a harmless outlet, the headache will usually vanish—until the next time.

The question is, while waiting for the headache to disappear, what can you do about it? Swallow an aspirin? Pop a tranquilizer? Perhaps, if you're a drinking man, you race to the bar for a fast one, even though you know that drugs or alcohol can have bad side effects. But, you figure, anything to cure that headache!

If you lived in rural England, however, you'd more likely boil equal parts of vinegar and water, and inhale the fumes. Or, with an ice-cold mixture, you would sponge your forehead, your temples, under the throat and back of the neck repeatedly, letting the liquid evaporate on the skin. You could also lie down and use the frigid mixture as a compress.

Better still, if you didn't mind looking like a wounded soldier, you'd go for an updated version of the same folk remedy. From an ordinary brown paper bag, you'd cut several strips the width of your forehead and long enough to cover the temples. After soaking them in pure vinegar, you'd lie down and place them, one atop the other, over the forehead. You'd either tape them down or wait for them to dry, forming a tight-fitting mold, and then you'd continue about your day's activities.

Vinegar, a popular food for cooking and dressings, forms the basis of a number of English rural headache remedies. Another of their compresses consists of two tablespoons of vinegar mixed with a two-cup pot of hops tea, applied warm to the forehead. Since hops tea is itself a nerve relaxant, added benefits are gained by drinking a cupful along with the compress.

Or try this treatment that I learned from a farmer in Hereford. Wash a handful of watercress, place it in a jar, and pour a pint of boiling vinegar over it. Cover and let steep for two hours. Strain, bottle, and refrigerate. Use on pads of cotton to sponge the temples and forehead or on a cloth as a compress.

Inhaling the scent of native vegetation has long been a popular folk remedy for tension headaches. The farmers of Andorra sniff crushed lemon verbena leaves, fresh or dried. Fresh hops and bruised fresh dill or dill seed are favorites among the Germans. Natives of the Spice Islands prefer the pungency of cloves or sage, while their kinsmen in the nearby Celebes inhale the heady aromas of bruised fresh peppermint or spearmint leaves. Inhabitants of Jaffa, Israel, take whiffs of fresh or dried orange peels, and Sicilian grove-tenders do the same with lemon peels. Spaniards recommend a remedy handed down by ancient Iberian tribes: fresh or dried betony rose leaves. Lavender buds and violets, also fresh or dried, are favored inhalants among the French.

Several of these remedies are available as oils. A California friend of mine carries her favorite mixture in a purse, to sniff as a smog-headache preventive. Into a tiny bottle with tight-fitting cork, she puts ten drops of lemon verbena oil, ten drops oil of peppermint, ten drops oil of lavender, five drops oil of cloves, and a few crushed anise seeds. A drop or two of the oils may be used separately, to rub on the forehead, temples, or back of the neck. And if fresh mint is available, the crushed, slightly dampened leaves make a refreshing, soothing compress for the forehead.

The Choctaw Indians pounded elder leaves and rubbed them on the head or, mixed with salt, applied them as a compress. Chickasaw tribesmen soaked small branches of cedar in water, and bound them around the head.

From the German Alsatians comes a charming headache remedy that seems to have particular appeal to women. Fill a quart jar half full of white rose petals, firmly packed. (White rose petals bring the best results, but if they're not available, red ones may be substituted.) Pour seventy percent rubbing alcohol over the petals till the jar is full, and let stand uncovered in the sun all day. If any alcohol evaporates, refill the jar, cover, and refrigerate. Use to rub on the forehead, temples, and neck or to dampen a cloth and apply as a compress.

In addition to their other healthful properties, many herb teas are natural nervines. Any of the following has a tranquilizing effect that soothes tensions and relieves headache pain:

angelica
balm (also known as lemon balm
    or sweet balm)
chamomile
feverfew
hops
lavender
marjoram

mint (peppermint or spearmint)
passion flower
rosemary
sage
sarsaparilla
vervain
Yerba santa

Civilized people seem to pride themselves on their exotic recipes and variegated menus. Their foods, "rich" in undigestible fats and nonnutritious carbohydrates, may be pleasing to the palate—but at the other end of the digestive tract, they often take a severe toll. As a result, two of modern man's commonest complaints are constipation and diarrhea.

Each native culture has its own specific food remedies for constipation. Adding them all together, we arrive at one general rule: *Eat plenty of fresh fruits and vegetables.*

Most fruits, leafy greens, and other low-starch vegetables supply a combination of moisture and bulk that help overcome irregularity. At least two servings of each should be included in the daily diet, preferably raw, unless you have an ulcer, colitis, or some similar ailment.

Here are the fruits that have been found most effective in improving elimination: Apples, pears, persimmons, pineapple (fresh), fresh and dried figs, and stewed rhubarb sweetened with honey. For best results, dried prunes and figs should not be cooked; pour boiling water over them and let them soak overnight. If sweetening is desired, stir honey into the boiling water before pouring it over the fruit. And don't pour out the water they're soaked in—drink it!

One or two tablespoonfuls of blackstrap molasses, before bedtime, is an excellent natural laxative from the Balkans. It's also a good source of important minerals, and is rich in the B vitamins, which help fight constipation by toning and strengthening the muscles of the intestinal tract.

If you don't like the taste of pure blackstrap molasses, stir it into a glass of milk, fruit juice, or water. And for extra laxative benefits, stir it into prune juice. Because it's a concentrated sweet, rinse your mouth or brush your teeth afterward.

Another healthful, concentrated sweet, with mild laxative properties, is honey. If its effects are too mild for you, try mixing it half and half with blackstrap molasses.

Buttermilk, clabber milk, kefir, and yogurt help destroy putrefactive bacteria in the intestinal tract, keeping it clean and healthy. Their lactic acid content promotes an increase in the "friendly" bacteria that fight off the "unfriendly" germs that invade the colon. And yogurt, in some mysterious way known only to itself, actually manufactures a supply of the B vitamins so essential to the health and strength of the intestinal tract and its muscles.

Just as any piece of machinery needs lubrication to keep it

running smoothly, so does your "food factory." Two or three tablespoonfuls each day of safflower, soybean, or other vegetable oil, can give your body's machinery the lubrication it needs to keep it unclogged and functioning efficiently. And surely you know the other health and nutritive benefits of these essential unsaturated oils.

I do as the Romans (and other Italians) do—I mix one of these oils with lemon juice or vinegar and herbs, to use as a salad dressing. If I couldn't do that, I'd take the oil straight by the spoonful.

From Byelorussia comes a natural food laxative made of steamed dried apples, honey, and yogurt. Even more effective is an added Ukranian touch: the same combination with shredded raw apple.

The Japanese have handed down two time-tested remedies for constipation: flaxseed (or linseed) and agar-agar. One was a favorite of their farmers; the other was preferred by their fishermen.

Flaxseed is a natural laxative that provides roughage and has a soothing, mucilaginous quality. It may be eaten raw, sprinkled over salads and cereals, cooked in cereal or mixed with milk or fruit juices. As a liquid, it should be drunk immediately, before it thickens. If it gets too thick to drink, just eat it with a spoon.

Agar-agar, the mineral-rich gelatine from seaweed, forms a smooth, slippery bulk in the intestines. This makes it an excellent natural laxative. The fishermen of Yokosuka combine it with fruit juice or fresh fruit, to make a gelatine salad or dessert, or they simply sprinkle it on fresh or stewed fruit.

Diarrhea, the opposite of constipation, may be a symptom of some more serious illness that requires professional diagnosis and treatment. But for mild cases, in which the stomach is rejecting some unsuitable food, a number of old-time remedies have proved successful.

In many Midwest locales, treatment consists of nothing more than several hours of fasting and a bowel-flushing enema as often as needed, until the cleansing of toxic wastes is complete. Liquids are taken, preferably warm, to replace the body's loss of fluid, but solid food is avoided until the stools return to normal.

Both American and English folk remedies include two time-tested specifics for diarrhea: boiled barley water and red raspberry leaf tea. British herbalists also recommend an old Scotch Highland remedy: a pinch of allspice stirred into a cup of warm water or milk.

If you're the adventurous type, and you own a fireplace, you might be intrigued by a quaint Welsh country standby. Place a red-hot poker in a cup of boiled milk for about thirty seconds, then drink the milk slowly. The theory is that the hot poker charges the milk with iron emanations, and iron is one of the homeopathic remedies for diarrhea. If nothing else, the boiled milk alone is beneficial for diarrhea.

Grated raw apple is an old European remedy that's still considered one of the best. But only the Russians give precise directions: one raw apple, peeled, cored, grated, or pureed, every two hours, with no other food or medication during the attack. Russian farmers also recommend teas brewed from raspberry leaf, linden flower, or sage.

Just as modern eating habits are responsible for many ailments, so too are some of the clothes we wear. Dressing in high style is bound to make you more attractive, but at what cost in comfort? Often an ache, pain, or growth can be traced to clothing that squeezes in the wrong places, cuts down blood circulation to parts of the body, and irritates sensitive, vulnerable areas.

In this connection, I'm reminded of a joint family outing we took with our friends, the Franklins. After a short hike through the woods, Chuck Franklin halted in pain and began massaging his foot.

"Lelord," he said despondently, "how do you go about preventing corns and calluses?"

Before I could reply, my eight-year-old grandson piped in, "Go barefoot!"

That was a hard answer to top. Under the demands of modern living, I could only give Chuck the "second best" solution: Wear shoes that are neither too tight nor too loose. I also gave Chuck a few treatments and preventives handed down through the ages.

In ancient India, where the castor bean first grew, Brahman physicians were the first to discover that castor oil, applied frequently to hard corns and calluses, relieves the soreness by keeping the tissue soft. When applied early enough, castor oil can stop formation of the corn—and, if used consistently, may even effect a cure.

Juice squeezed from the stem of a dandelion, and applied to the corn, has been called a "sure cure" by sheepherders of Australia. British herbalists claim the same results from the juice of a herbaceous plant, celandine (sometimes called white bryony or tetterwort), but dandelion is a lot easier to come by. Several applications of dandelion juice may be necessary, but two of celandine are usually considered enough.

An eighteenth-century Bavarian remedy for corns is to take the yeast of beer, spread it on a clean cloth and bind the cloth over the corn. If the application is renewed every day, a cure is said to take place within three or four weeks. If you don't like beer, try substituting that remarkable food supplement, brewer's yeast (a by-product of brewing). Moisten it with lemon juice, spread on absorbent cotton, and bind the cotton over the corn.

Many Russians soak a small piece of their famous black bread in vinegar and bind it to the corn. Another of their old folk-remedies is a poultice made by mixing bicarbonate of soda and castor oil.

The Osage Indians used to bind bruised ivy leaves on corns and calluses. Later, when vinegar was available to them, they soaked the ivy leaves in vinegar overnight and wore the poultice during the day, repeating the treatment until relief was obtained. For the prevention and relief of sore, burning feet, Tunica tribesmen lined the bottoms of their moccasins with fresh alder leaves.

A slice of lemon bound to a corn, and left on overnight, is an old Sicilian remedy. Repeat the treatment as often as necessary, using a fresh slice of lemon each night.

Perhaps even more effective is a Polynesian remedy: fresh pineapple, thinly sliced or grated, bound to the corn in the same way as lemon. But it must be *fresh* pineapple, not canned. Cooking kills the enzymes and decreases the acid content, and both enzymes and acid are an essential part of this treatment.

British herbalists recommend preparing your feet for both these applications by first soaking them in a basin of hot water with a half cup of Epsom salts dissolved in it. If you don't have Epsom salts, use bicarbonate of soda. Both help relieve soreness, burning, and inflammation.

Another common ailment, which strikes mostly the aged, is

dropsy, or edema. Caused by abnormal accumulation of fluid in the tissues, resulting in painful swelling, dropsy is not a disease in itself. It is usually the symptom of another disease or a dietary deficiency (especially a low-protein, high-carbohydrate diet), or it can result from an injury.

Inhabitants of the Japanese coast treat the condition with ground kelp, which stimulates the kidneys to eliminate excess water. Kelp, by the way, is now available in most countries as granules or tablets.

Dwellers in the Australian outback dig up the roots of the dock plant, boil them, and drink the water. In some parts of rural America, especially the South, a tea brewed from mullein leaves has long been considered one of the best remedies for dropsy.

The diuretic (kidney-flushing) properties of steamed fresh asparagus (and the water it's cooked in) are well known among asparagus eaters of all countries. The same is true of parsley tea or parsley and milk.

When dropsy is caused by a dietary deficiency, increase the amount of protein and calcium in the diet and cut down drastically on carbohydrates, which hold both salt and water in the tissues. Season with herb and kelp granules instead of salt. One of the B-vitamins, pantothenic acid, increases the excretion of salt and helps reduce the swelling.

A cardiac condition and kidney disease are other causes of dropsy, but they require professional treatment.

With the spread of smog and other forms of air pollution, tired or inflamed eyes have become one of modern society's most common ailments. Simple eye fatigue and mild inflammation can be helped by any number of folk remedies.

In parts of India, inflamed eyes and reddened eyelids are still treated with a drop of castor oil placed in the eyes and applied to the edge of the lids. If you ever try this remedy yourself, be sure to use a fresh bottle of castor oil, not one that's been opened long enough to become rancid.

A drop or two of pure honey in the eyes is an old Vermont remedy. English beekeepers recommend a less sticky way of using honey: Add three tablespoonfuls of honey to two cups of boiling water, and stir until the honey is thoroughly dissolved. Allow to cool, then bathe the eyes with it several times a day.

Or moisten pads of absorbent cotton with it, and use as a soothing, healing compress.

If you have access to sea salt, you might like to duplicate a natural eyewash handed down by ancient Cornish seafarers. Let a pint of water stand overnight in an uncovered glass jar, to allow the chlorine to escape from it. Bring the water to a boil, add two level teaspoonfuls of sea salt, and stir to dissolve thoroughly. Cool and pour into a sterilized bottle or jar. Keep tightly covered.

For tired bloodshot eyes and itchy, reddened eyelids, Taiwanese farmers moisten tea bags in boiling water, allow them to cool to a comfortable temperature, and apply them as a compress. When an irritation results in a sty, the farmers bring it to a head and ease the soreness and speed its healing with hot tea-bag compresses.

An Irish remedy for sties and inflammation is a poultice made by steaming fresh cabbage leaves in boiling water until heated through and slightly limp, but not cooked. Drain and apply the leaves warm to the eyes. Another sore-eye healer from Ireland is a poultice made of scraped raw potato.

The benefits of the cabbage-leaf poultice were discovered long ago by Hollywood. It was standard treatment for actors afflicted with "Kleig eyes," a condition in which eyes become inflamed and bloodshot. It was caused by the intense glare of the lights used in the early days of motion pictures.

American Indians relied on a variety of herbs to clear and strengthen sore, inflamed eyes. Mesquite, blue flax leaves, sassafras root, red maple leaves, and other plants were dried, reduced to a powder, and made into a salve or steeped in boiling water to make an eyewash or lotion.

Two well-known Blackfoot lotions were made by pouring boiling water over sesame leaves or the leaves and flowers of yarrow. Allowed to steep, then cooled, both were used to bathe the eyes or to moisten a cloth for a compress.

The herb eyebright, according to naturopaths, is a useful remedy for all eye ailments, including conjunctivitis and ulcers. Culpeper, in one of his grandiose moments, described it as "a restorer of failing sight." And, he continued, "If eyebright were as much used as it is neglected, it would have spoilt the trade of the spectacle-makers."

In England a strong eye lotion is made (for external use only) by steeping a handful of the whole eyebright plant in a pint of water, and using it on cotton pads as a compress. American herbalists prefer an eyewash made of equal parts of chamomile and eyebright, steeped in boiling water and strained through a sterilized cloth.

While you are experimenting with remedies, it is important to remember that even a mild deficiency of vitamin A can cause poor night vision, eyes that tire easily, and susceptibility to such infections as sties, corneal ulcers, iritis, and conjunctivitis. Vitamin B-2 deficiency may produce burning, watering, reddening and itching of the eyes, sensitivity to light, and blurred or dim vision. That is why both these vitamins have been used successfully in treating corneal ulcers.

Tired eyes will also benefit by resting them frequently, bathing them in cold water, or applying a cold, wet compress for a few minutes. Closing the eyes and rolling them to the extreme right and left, then up and down, will help relieve eyestrain. So will closing the eyes and massaging gently in a circular motion over the eyeball with the middle finger.

May I be so bold as to add my personal contribution to the lore of folk remedies? This recipe combines a number of foods essential for eye-health, which is why I call it the . . .

Lelord Kordel "Bright-Eyes Cocktail"

1 cup orange juice	1 tablespoon brewer's yeast
1 cup fresh carrot juice	flakes
1 teaspoon rose hips powder	3 tablespoons wheat germ
¼ cup powdered skim milk	¼ cup sunflower seeds
1 egg yolk	honey to taste

Combine in an electric blender until all ingredients are well mixed. Makes two generous servings. If no blender is available, omit the sunflower seeds and stir thoroughly or shake in a jar.

The biological "dues" we pay for eating the wrong foods is nowhere more evident than in the mass of advertising that surrounds cures for simple indigestion. There are liquids that "coat" the stomach with a protective lining, pills that "neutralize" fifty times their weight in excess acid, powders that "soothe" the nerves of an overactive digestive tract.

What none of the ads mentions is that persistent indigestion, lasting over a period of time, may be a symptom of some serious disease requiring professional treatment. And, of course, it's bad business to admit that minor attacks, caused by eating the wrong foods—especially when under pressure—can be relieved by a change of diet, a change of pace, and one of several simple home remedies.

The same is true of peptic indigestion, which results from an insufficiency of hydrochloric acid. Without hydrochloric acid, your stomach can't digest protein foods properly, and the absorption of protein, vitamins, and minerals is impaired. In most persons, the stomach acids that digest proteins tend to decrease steadily after maturity. Unless a suitable substitute is found for those suffering from a deficiency, peptic ulcer will remain something to be endured instead of cured.

Throughout France it is common practice to drink a small glass of dry wine before dinner. This aids digestion and protein absorption by increasing the flow of the digestive enzymes. For French teetotalers, hot vegetable broth does the same job.

In the Balkans, where lactic acid foods are virtual staples of the diet, indigestion rarely occurs. Lactic acid is an excellent substitute for hydrochloric acid—so at the first sign of stomach trouble, the natives increase their consumption of sauerkraut.

Oatmeal and okra are two remedies from the American Southland. Both have a demulcent quality that protects the sensitive duodenal surfaces and soothes the stomach and intestines.

Herbal teas that have been found especially beneficial for calming a nervous stomach and relieving digestive upsets, are fenugreek, angelica, lemon balm, chamomile, catnip, comfrey, dandelion, hops, papaya, peppermint, sage, and valerian.

Most connoisseurs of herbal tea like to experiment with all varieties until they find the flavors they like best and those that benefit them the most. For extra benefits, they often try two or more in combination. Papaya and mint are favorite go-togethers in the tropics. Middle Europeans lean toward comfrey and hops, while Britishers prefer chamomile or papaya tea with two or three drops of essence of peppermint added to each cup.

Mediterraneans seem to prefer equal parts of hops and sage tea steeped with one half teaspoonful of anise seed.

The American Indians had many plant remedies for stomach distress. Two that are still widely used, both here and in Europe, are dandelion and ginger root. The Iroquois used to dig the roots from the earth, then wash and boil them into a strong decoction. To the dandelion brew, they added a few leaves for additional tonic properties.

A long-revered Aztec remedy, still used in Mexico, combines the unique talents of three teas. Damiana leaves are an ancient nerve tonic. Chamomile soothes the nerves and increases the flow of digestive juices. Anise seeds relieve flatulence, the painful condition caused by gas in the stomach and bowels. Brew equal parts together, to ease nervous stomach and indigestion and to calm the nerves under pressure.

The Soviet Tatars drink four ounces of goat's milk three times a day as an aid to digestion, especially when the symptoms are heartburn and belching.

For fast relief from the pain of flatulence, Norwegians simmer one teaspoonful of dill seeds in a glass of water for twenty minutes. While the liquid is still hot, they strain and drink it.

Corsican farmers prefer a flavorful remedy made by simmering one tablespoonful each of anise seed and honey in a glass of water for fifteen minutes. Dose: two tablespoonfuls of the strained liquid before each meal.

The Irish put their faith in a few sprigs of fresh mint leaves steeped in a pot of tea. When available, three or four birch buds are added to the brew or used instead of mint.

In Bolivia the Amerindian natives use an infusion of cloves. A cup of boiling water poured over five or six cloves, and allowed to steep, covered, for several minutes, acts to eliminate excess gas in the stomach and intestines, and relieve pain and distention. Cloves also help promote the flow of gastric juices and improve the digestion.

Chinese legend has it that leaves picked from their tea plants, just after the first thunderstorm of the year, make a brew of exceptional medicinal quality. In particular, they recommend a tea brewed from their wonder plant, ginseng, as a remedy for stomach and digestive disorders.

Perhaps more than any other nation, England has been the

source of folk treatments now being used in America and other parts of the world. The following seed and plant remedies are only a few of the many we've borrowed from her.

Caraway julep: Bruise an ounce of caraway seeds, place them in a jar, and pour a pint of boiling water over them. Cover tightly and let stand overnight. The next day, strain and bottle. A tablespoonful, taken whenever there are symptoms of nervous indigestion and flatulence, will ease pain, soothe the digestive tract, and relieve distention.

Chamomile tea with allspice: Along with cloves and several other spices, allspice is classed by herbalists as a stomachic and a carminative, which means it's an agent used to relieve colic, gripping, and flatulence. To one cup of chamomile tea, sweetened with honey, if desired, add one-eighth teaspoonful of allspice.

Coriander seeds: Also classed as a carminative, both the seeds and leaves of coriander have long been known as excellent stomach remedies. The leaves, when available, may be mixed with salad greens. Dose: one-half teaspoonful of seeds mixed with honey and eaten before meals. Or steep the same amount of seeds in a cup of your favorite tea, and drink it three times a day, preferably half an hour before meals.

Hops tea with mustard seed: For hundreds of years, mustard seed has been a European aid to digestion and a remedy for intestinal and digestive disorders. Add one-half teaspoonful of seeds to a cup of hops tea and take twice a day, half an hour before meals for severe cases, or the same amount, as needed, for an occasional upset. For best results, the seeds should be swallowed whole with the tea, not chewed.

Ginger-mint julep: To make this remedy with the delicious-sounding name, add one-eighth teaspoonful of powdered ginger to a cup of mint tea and sweeten with honey to taste. If you like, add a slice of lemon.

Marjoram: According to an old-time herbalist named Gerarde, marjoram "may be used to good purpose by those who cannot brook their meate, and is very good against the wambling of the stomach."

I haven't heard of many "wambling" stomach complaints lately, but marjoram is a versatile plant that has a long record of treating a variety of ailments. The early Romans used it as a tea to "strengthen the brain, nerves, and stomach." Though I can't vouch for its effect on the brain, I do know that it's a well-known remedy for nervous indigestion and sour stomach.

The British drink marjoram tea for nervous indigestion and headaches. When fresh marjoram is available, they add a sprinkling of the chopped leaves to salads or make a sandwich by placing a few sprigs between two slices of buttered whole-grain bread.

Of course, the best preventive "medicine" of all is a sensible diet. Your stomach was made for simple, natural meals, high in protein, fresh vegetables, and fruit and low in sugar and starch. In addition, if you don't overload your stomach and do try to eat when you're relaxed, you should be able to avoid most of the digestive complaints prevalent in today's society.

Such a diet will also aid in improving the function of the vital organs of the body that hold the key to your chances for a long and healthy life. Two organs subject to mild, treatable ailments are the kidneys and liver. Knowing how to keep these important organs in good condition, and what to do for minor ailments as soon as they occur, will give you a better chance of avoiding the serious illnesses that require special treatment.

To keep the kidneys and bladder healthy, or to remedy mild inflammation and other minor disorders, New Englanders rely on two of their time-tested staples: honey and apple cider vinegar. They also believe in including an abundance of asparagus, carrots, kidney beans, and parsnips in the diet, and in drinking plenty of cranberry juice and lemonade.

The amount of food and fruit juices needed to get results seems to vary with each individual. As one native of Cape Cod told me, "We let our conscience, size, and appetite be our guide." He admitted, however, that New England doctors advise an eight-ounce glass of cranberry juice three times a day for kidney inflammation and a glass of lemonade "as often as you feel like it, or oftener."

More precise is a British home-℞ that calls for twenty-five stalks of washed asparagus, cut into inch-long pieces. Place in a large saucepan and cover with a quart of water. Bring to a boil, lower heat, cover, and simmer slowly until the liquid is reduced to half. Cool and strain through a cloth, squeezing well. Dose: a tablespoonful of the decoction every four hours.

Melons are high on the list of foods that are cleansing and beneficial to the kidneys—with watermelon at the top. A tea made by simmering watermelon seed in water for thirty minutes has been a favorite kidney and bladder remedy for hundreds of years. A combination of the tea and fresh watermelon is considered even more effective. In the winter, when watermelons aren't available, pumpkinseed tea may be substituted.

In India, the tropical fruit, mango, has long been used to treat nephritis, an inflammation of the kidneys. Other fruits and vegetables used in their native habitats to treat ailing kidneys, are apples, pears, nectarines, blackberries, green beans, beets and beet greens, mustard greens, cabbage, carrots, celery, summer squash and parsley, kale, turnip greens, watercress, dandelion greens.

In England, several herb teas are drunk regularly as "tonic for the kidneys." Among the most popular are strawberry, dandelion, sassafras, comfrey, and a tea made from the leaves and blooms of wild carrot.

Many of the remedies for kidney complaints are the same that have proved beneficial in liver disorders. When you realize that the failure of the kidneys to eliminate poisons will eventually cause liver damage, you can readily understand the correlation between these organs. The liver itself does a good job of eliminating poisons and toxins circulating in the body, but with environmental pollution at an all-time high, it might need a little help from its friends in the medicinal food kingdom.

A Russian remedy for cleansing and stimulating the liver is a daily cup of beet juice. In England, a favorite liver cleanser and detoxifier combines three ounces of carrot juice, three of beet juice, and two of celery juice. The Irish chop a small head of lettuce, simmer it in a quart of water for twenty minutes, strain it, and take two tablespoonfuls every hour.

Australians rely upon a combination of herb teas—equal parts of dandelion and hops. Other herbs that benefit the liver are agrimony, angelica, cleavers, comfrey, and goldenseal.

In France, where they seem to have more than their share of

liver complaints, a diet of nothing but water and eight ounces of apple juice, every two hours, is followed for one or two days. On the morning after the final day of dieting, breakfast consists of one eight-ounce glass of apple juice followed by four ounces of olive oil.

From Panama comes a refreshing and pleasant-tasting remedy that I'd enjoy whether it made my liver happy or not. It's made by squeezing two or three limes in a glass of water and sweetening to taste with honey. Recommended dosage: as much as you can take. That shouldn't be difficult, especially on a hot day!

For the final remedy in this category, I've saved an easy, anatomy-shaking liver activator that doesn't cost a cent. It comes from a British herbalist, Mary Thorne Quelch, who quotes a London specialist in liver disorders: "People who are 'liverish' would benefit to an extraordinary degree if they cultivated a really good laugh every morning before setting foot out of their bedrooms."

A hearty laugh not only shakes and activates the liver. It aids the digestion, exercises the diaphragm, and expands the lungs. This, in turn, benefits the heart and just about all the other organs and glands in the body.

It's a good way to start the day. Why not try it? Even if at first you have nothing to laugh at but yourself!

WORLDWIDE REMEDIES
FOR EVERYDAY AILMENTS

Edema
(Dropsy)

Potato Peeling Tea—From Ireland

Handful of potato peelings, well washed
2 cups water

Scrub potatoes thoroughly before peeling. Place peelings in a saucepan and cover with water. Bring to a boil, reduce heat and simmer slowly, covered for twenty minutes. Strain.

Dose: Two tablespoonfuls in a glass of water four times a day.

Treatment can be continued as long as necessary, but it is reported that after a few days of treatment the swelling disappears and legs and ankles regain their normal size.

Dandelion Root-Juniper Berry Decoction—From Holland

½ ounce dandelion root, well scrubbed
1 quart cold water
½ ounce juniper berries, bruised

Put dandelion root and water in a saucepan and bring to a boil. Cover and simmer slowly until liquid is reduced to a pint. Place juniper berries in a jar and pour boiling mixture over them. Let stand until cool, then strain.

Variation: If dried broom tops are available, add ½ ounce to the jar of juniper berries for a more potent diuretic.

Parsley-Milk—From Russia

2 pounds parsley, washed and chopped
1 quart unpasteurized milk

Place parsley in glass or enamel casserole and pour milk over it. Place casserole in a slow oven until about half of the liquid has evaporated. Cool and strain.

Dose: One to two tablespoons every two hours.

Note: This is a powerful diuretic and should not be taken more than two or three days a week.

Indigestion
Home Remedy for Peptic Indigestion—From New England

1 tablespoon cider vinegar
1 tablespoon honey
1 cup hot water

Mix ingredients and stir until honey dissolves.

Dose: Sip slowly, preferably twenty or thirty minutes before meals.

Digestive Aid—From Germany

1 teaspoon ground hops
1 tablespoon glycerine
1 cup boiling water

Place hops in scalded teapot. Add glycerine and water and stir. Cover and let steep for five minutes. Strain and drink one half hour before meals.

Kordel Variation: Substitute one cup of freshly brewed hops tea for the ground hops and add one teaspoonful honey. Drink one half hour before meals.

Kidney Tonics
Flaxseed-Lemon Decoction—From Russia

4 tablespoons flaxseed
1 quart water
juice of 1 lemon

Simmer flaxseed in water for ten minutes. Cool and add lemon juice. Thin mixture to a more desirable consistency by adding warm water, or eat it by the spoonful.

Dose: one half cup every two hours for two consecutive days or as needed.

Apple-Honey Tea—From Ireland

3 or 4 apples
honey

Wash apples well, but do not peel. Slice. Place in a pan lined with oiled parchment and dry slowly in a low oven with the door open. When thoroughly dried, close oven and roast until apple slices are well browned. Store in a dry place. To use, place a few slices in a teapot, pour boiling water over them and steep for six to eight minutes. Sweeten with honey.

Dose: two or three cups a day or as needed.

Four-Herb Kidney Remedy—From England

1 ounce asparagus root
1 ounce celery root
1 ounce fennel
1 ounce parsley root
1 pint water
lemon juice

Place roots in a clean jar with a lid and pour boiling water over them. Allow to stand overnight.

Dose: Four ounces of the liquid with a few drops of lemon juice before each meal, for two or three consecutive days. Repeat every three or four months for what the British call "the best insurance against kidney disease now and in later years."

Laxatives
Agaragar and Flaxseed (or Linseed)—From Japan

> 1 pint boiling water
> 1 ounce agaragar
> 1 teaspoon flaxseed (or linseed)

Add agaragar and flaxseed to boiling water. Simmer slowly for about five minutes. Cool and take one or two teaspoonfuls of the jellied substance before each meal.

For a tastier variation: Substitute fruit juice for the boiling water.

Herbal Fruit Laxative—From Australia

> ½ pound prunes, cooked
> ½ pound figs, cooked
> 1 cup dark molasses, preferably blackstrap
> 1 pint water
> 1 ounce senna tea or dried leaves

Remove stones from prunes and chop prunes and figs coursely. Add dark molasses and tea made by steeping senna leaves in boiling water. Allow to stand twenty minutes before straining. Combine all ingredients and simmer until the fruit is reduced to a soft consistency. Cool and spoon into jars.

Dose: one or two tablespoonfuls at bedtime for adults; more if needed. *For children: two teaspoonfuls.*

Natural Laxative—From Bulgaria

> 1 cup yogurt
> 5 prunes, chopped
> 2 tablespoons blackstrap molasses

Stir until ingredients are well mixed. For a smooth maltlike consistency, mix in an electric blender.

Dose: At bedtime, for breakfast, or both.

5

Remedies Old and Updated, for Aches and Pains

How often we see it on television. A bleary-eyed man lies in bed, choking and wheezing, moaning hoarsely to his wife that they'll have to cancel an important dinner date tonight. Nonsense, replies his wife, smiling with confidence as she plies him with a spoonful of syrup.

Or is it an antihistamine pill that she feeds him? Or maybe aspirin in one of its numerous varieties? Whatever the product being touted, a fast turn of the clock brings our couple to their dinner destination, the husband bright-eyed and bushy-tailed, marveling at the resourceful spouse who came up with such a quick-acting cold remedy.

How about the distraught housewife who's about to explode because the children are making too much racket or her mother-in-law added too much salt to the soup? Swiftly she moves to the medicine cabinet, where she downs a couple of tranquilizers. Lo and behold, her tension headache vanishes so rapidly that the kids' screaming sounds like violins and the ruined soup tastes like an Escoffier creation.

Then, of course, there are portrayals of numerous antacids for the overindulgent eater, laxatives for irregularity, salves or liniments for aching joints, supergermicides for scrapes, cuts, and bruises. Thanks to the long list of "ethical" pharmaceutical products, the examples are legion. They all add up to one fact: In the endless war between modern science and ancient folk remedies, the biggest battle is taking place in your own home.

Unfortunately, the conflict is one-sided. Against the vast financial resources of the drug manufacturers and their hand-maidens, the advertising agencies, how can the herbalists hope to compete? The average consumer, bombarded with promises of miraculous recoveries on TV and radio, in newspapers and magazines, is rarely exposed to the advantages of natural healing. More important, he is barred from learning the built-in risks of patent medicines.

Not only are many of the highly advertised products over-priced and ineffective, but often a key ingredient of the medication is a drug that can produce harmful side effects. According to the head of one bureau for consumer protection, "There are hundreds of thousands of hospital admissions every year resulting from adverse reactions to over-the-counter drugs."

The same cannot be said of nature's remedies, whether used for serious internal disorders or for the simplest of everyday ailments and injuries. Speaking on the subject of bites, stings, cuts, and burns, Dr. Peter N. Horvath, chief of dermatology at Georgetown University Medical Center, declared, "The problem with many of the drugstore remedies is that some people are allergic to them."

Dr. Horvath's statement reflects a growing awareness in the scientific community of the debt owed by modern pharmacology to the wisdom of the ancient herbalists and so-called folk-healers. For these pioneers have supplied modern science with remarkable data which, when subjected to laboratory scrutiny, do indeed prove that food and flower remedies are more than matters of blind faith.

Case history: Robert Marsh, a worker in a manufacturing firm in Lehigh Valley in Pennsylvania, suffered massive burns in a plant explosion. Doctors warned him that it would take at least six months for the burns to heal, that several skin grafts would be necessary to replace destroyed tissue, and that he'd probably never regain full use of his right arm, hand, and fingers.

Two days later, back home, Robert Marsh's wife, Carol, began home treatment with alpha-tocopherol vitamin E. She squeezed the contents of two capsules into an antibiotic ointment and started a regular schedule of dressing his burns with it. In addition, she gave him a vitamin E capsule of two hundred units, three times a day.

Less than a week after the accident, Robert Marsh visited a plastic surgeon to prepare for the series of skin grafts. The surgeon, amazed at the healing that had taken place, told him that no grafts were necessary and that he should continue with his present treatment.

What do the known healing properties of vitamin E have to do with folk medicine? One clue comes from an old German burn remedy consisting of *honey, comfrey leaves, and wheat germ oil,* which is rich in vitamin E. This recipe, which appears at the end of the chapter, may be too complicated for the average homemaker to dabble with, but it does coincide with an easier modern burn ointment that has proved effective: *Simply puncture and squeeze the contents of some alpha-tocopherol vitamin E capsules into a jar of petroleum jelly (Vaseline).*

The notion of concocting homemade remedies, based on age-old recipes, is not as farfetched as it seems. If your household contains such common products as turpentine (derived from the longleaf pine), witch hazel (extracted from the plant of the same name), and camphor (from the camphor tree), you already have some of nature's ingredients on hand. Add to these the wealth of beneficial foods at your disposal, and you are already equipped with elements of ancient and modern folk remedies that are safe, economical, and remarkably effective when used as prescribed. In the words of Dr. Horvath, "It's very unlikely that anyone will be allergic to vinegar, sour cream, cooking oil, oatmeal, and other kitchen remedies that have proved effective."

A famous "kitchen remedy" handed down by the American Indian consists of *two parts of sunflower seed oil and one part turpentine, mixed thoroughly and used as a liniment.* Easy to prepare, it reportedly works wonders when rubbed on sprains and sore muscles.

Another Indian recipe for the same condition was *witch hazel bark simmered in sunflower oil or set in the sun, uncovered, for several days.* Think of the time they would have saved if distilled witch hazel were readily available to them, as it is to you at your local drugstore!

From Italian antiquity comes an equally effective homemade remedy for sprains and sore muscles: *a combination of half camphor and half olive oil.* It is still in use in many parts of Italy.

A Russian folk remedy for sprains and pulled ligaments consists of two kitchen ingredients: *finely chopped onion mixed with honey and used as a poultice.*

Another effective liniment, from England, combines four household products: *equal parts of sunflower seed oil, oil of turpentine, oil of camphor, and oil of cloves.* One part oil of wintergreen is optional, but it makes a soothing, pleasant-smelling addition. This combination is used not only for sprains, but as a rub for muscle spasms and rheumatic and arthritic pains.

Also from England comes a rub for sprains, sore muscles, and rheumatic pains that dates back to the eleventh century: *rosemary leaves boiled in oil.*

Any survey of folk healing, modern or ancient, quickly reveals that each society makes use of whatever foods and plants are available. Over the centuries, every culture experimented with—and perfected—whatever "tools" it had on hand.

Hence the inhabitants of Bulgaria, the land of yogurt and other lactic acid foods, have their own unique remedy for sprains, strains, and sore or pulled muscles: *a compress of hot soured milk or buttermilk.* This is applied directly to the injury, with frequent fresh applications.

Gypsies, since time immemorial, have lived off a multitude of roots and flowers. So it's no surprise that a well-known Hungarian gypsy ointment is made from *a cupful of marigolds simmered in a cupful of lard.*

Depending on the time and care you wish to give yourself, "kitchen treatments" range from the utterly simple to the complicated. An old English folk remedy, for injured bones and muscles, uses *vinegar* in two different ways:

1. Moisten a flannel cloth with vinegar and place it over the injury. Take a hot iron and glide it over the cloth till the congestion and pain are "ironed out."

2. Dip a strip of brown paper in vinegar until it's moistened thoroughly (but not till it falls apart). Wrap it snugly around the injured part, patting it gently but firmly to hold it in place. As it dries, it hardens into a homemade cast that gives support to the weakened area. When stronger support is needed, use several layers of vinegar-moistened paper, applied one at a time, with each strip pressed over the other to form a solid layer as they dry. When ready to renew, just peel the "cast" from the skin and apply a fresh one.

Among the commonest minor injuries are insect bites and stings, for which Dr. Horvath declared, "Your refrigerator and kitchen shelves hold a better selection of remedies than the corner drugstore." His research led the eminent dermatologist to this conclusion: *"Best for bites is meat tenderizer,* and it should be rubbed on the bite as soon as possible. In a few minutes, it will neutralize the poison."

This reminds me of the day I was stung by a sea nettle, while staying at a seaside hotel. There were no known kitchen remedies handy, but fresh papaya was available. Remembering that most meat tenderizers are made from papaya, I took a slice of the fresh fruit and bound it on the sting. Within minutes the poison seemed to be neutralized, the pain subsided, the swelling went down, healing began, and . . . *fresh papaya was added to my list of home remedies!*

When the body is covered with mosquito, chigger, or other insect bites, Dr. Horvath makes this recommendation: *a cupful or two of quick starch or minute oatmeal (or both) stirred into your bathwater.* "When you get into the tub," he says, "it's as good as covering your body with a solution of calamine lotion." If a bathtub is not available, try an application of *oatmeal and water made into a paste.*

In the absence of oatmeal or starch, a favorite old-time remedy is to sponge chigger bites with *kerosene-moistened cotton.* And tobacco growers, the world over, swear by this remedy: *moistened tobacco or its leaves placed on the bite.*

Bee and wasp stings can sometimes prove more complicated. Before you apply any treatment, the insect's stinger should be removed from the skin as soon as possible and ice cubes applied immediately, to numb the pain and relieve the swelling. Afterward, *baking soda, cider vinegar, or rubbing alcohol* make good applications. So does a combination of *baking soda, vinegar, and salt, made into a paste.* Three other folk remedies of proven value are *honey, liquid laundry bluing, or a wet compress of a few drops of household ammonia diluted in a cupful of water.*

Always remember, however, that these remedies apply only to minor injuries. If there is general collapse, excessive swelling, or other indications that the victim is allergic to bee or wasp stings, call a doctor at once.

Of course, there is no better protection against injury or illness than the proverbial "ounce of prevention." A healthy, well-rounded diet may not scare bees away or keep an ankle from twisting, but it can go a long way toward easing pain and speeding recovery. Burns, for example, are purely accidental, but, as in the case of Robert Marsh, there is much evidence that their intensity can be reduced and their healing accelerated by a diet rich in vitamin E.

Most of us have experienced first-degree burns at one time or another in our lives. These are the minor burns that extend only to the top layers of the skin, and they usually require only a mild application to soothe and relieve the reddened skin and to keep it from drying out. Whatever substance you use, it should be applied promptly.

Bicarbonate of soda and cold water, made into a paste, is a famous old-time remedy for minor burns. So are *petroleum jelly* and other mild ointments. *Margarine, butter, lard* or other cooking grease make fine applications. Better still are the *vegetable cooking oils* or *wheat germ oil* with its vitamin E content.

Thick cream or *rich top milk* are still widely used by dairy farmers. For city dwellers who have a hard time getting un-homogenized milk, Dr. Horvath suggests an available substitute. *"Sour cream,"* he says, "is an excellent, soothing medication that I recommend for small burns."

Second-degree burns, which extend deeper into the skin, should immediately be placed under cold running water for ten or fifteen minutes and gently cleansed with mild soap. Afterward, a sterile gauze dressing should be applied. Since these burns frequently cause great loss of fluids, the victim should replace his bodily supply by drinking lots of water or other liquids.

Third-degree burns extend to the deepest skin layer, called the corium. They must be examined at a hospital or by a doctor, as soon as possible. If immediate professional treatment is not available, the victim, while waiting, should keep the burned area under cold running water while drinking large quantities of fluids.

Another condition, in which all-around diet may be sig-nificant, is boils. Frequent outbreaks of boils could be a symp-tom of diabetes, and for that condition you should consult a professional. But in the majority of cases, boils are a sign that your body has a low resistance to infection. By improving your diet, you can build up your resistance.

To prevent boils, herbalists recommend such blood-purifying teas as *red clover, nettle,* and *sassafras,* taken twice a day. Another old-fashioned blood-purifier is a combination of *dark molasses and powdered flowers of sulphur.*

You can improve your blood by adding to your diet liver, beef, beef-tongue, apricots, leafy greens, parsley, and other iron-rich foods, including dark molasses. The blood-cleansing benefits of sulphur are also available in cabbage, Brussels sprouts, broccoli, and turnips.

If you do have a boil, an old English remedy utilizes the skin of hard-boiled eggs to relieve soreness and draw out infection. Carefully peel off the thin, membranous covering, moisten it and apply to the boil. Leave it on until the drawing process begins; change the application when it becomes soiled.

The Irish have handed down one of the most novel home-remedies for boils. Simply heat a bottle or small-mouthed jar by filling it with boiling water. Let it stand a few seconds, to heat thoroughly, then pour out the water and quickly put the mouth of the bottle over the boil. Hold it there until it cools. This creates a suction that will draw out the core when the bottle is removed.

American Indians used a variety of poultices and herbal remedies. Each tribe seemed to have its favorite, but among the most effective ones, easy to obtain, are poultices of crushed, ground, or lightly steamed violet or wild pansy leaves, catnip leaves, ground flaxseed, steamed yarrow, or wild dock leaves. Most of these are available, dried, in health food stores and herb shops. For best results, apply them warm.

If any or all of these remedies are unappealing or troublesome to you, there's one surefire "homegrown" treatment that's as easy as heating a pot of water. Because that's all it takes to make hot soaks or compresses. Hot water, applied to the infection, helps it come to a head more rapidly. The heat also increases circulation, expands the blood vessels, and speeds up the march of white blood cells to destroy the invading germs.

If the boil is on your hand, foot, posterior, or other soakable part of your body, immerse it in a basin of hot water. If not, apply hot, wet compresses.

For faster relief from soreness and inflammation, you might take a lead from some of the famous health spas around the world. Their healing, mineral-rich waters (called hypertonic solutions) can be re-created in your kitchen by dissolving either *plain salt, epsom salts, or boric acid in hot water*. The recipe for a more effective hypertonic solution appears at the end of this chapter.

The area around a boil or other infection should be cleansed several times daily, to keep the infection from spreading. One of the easiest ways is to moisten a cotton swab with rubbing alcohol and wipe off the entire area surrounding the boil. Painting around it with iodine works, too, and it's reported that swabbing the boil itself with iodine two or three times a day, when it first appears as a lump under the skin, will effect a cure before it gets a head start.

Other germicidal cleansings include a daily bath with an antiseptic surgical soap (available at your pharmacy without a prescription) and washing your hands thoroughly before touching the boil or the skin surrounding it.

And bear in mind one cardinal rule: *Never squeeze a boil!* By doing so, you increase the chances of spreading the infection and bruising the skin.

Bruises, too, may be the result of a dietary deficiency. Sometimes referred to as "black-and-blue marks," they occur when an injury ruptures the small blood vessels (capillaries) under the skin, causing internal bleeding.

If you bruise easily and often, the regular use of vitamin C and the bioflavonoids will help strengthen the capillaries. So will a folk recipe from Germany, consisting of *lemon and water,* which also appears at the end of this chapter.

Once you do get a black eye or other type of bruise (and inflammations, too), you might improvise a treatment which early American settlers learned from the Mohawk Indians. It was a decoction brewed from *witch hazel bark and leaves.*

The best treatment, however, is still the old-time remedy recommended by many doctors: *ice-cold compresses* or *ice cubes wrapped in a dampened washcloth or small Turkish towel,* applied immediately. Bruises more than a few hours old won't be helped by this treatment, but early applications will reduce pain and swelling and speed the healing process.

If ice cubes are used, keep the application on for about twenty minutes, then take it off for a few minutes. Repeat this procedure for about an hour or two.

While proper diet can go a long way toward protecting you against burns, boils, and bruises, there is one organism lurking around us which no amount of healthy eating can ward off. It is called *fungus,* and it seeks out warm, dark, moist places: between the toes, under and around the toenails, on the arms, legs, and in the outer ear.

The toe-thriving fungus known as athlete's foot is one of the most persistent species and also the most contagious. It is usually picked up around swimming pools, locker rooms, and other public places where people walk barefooted. From there, it is easily transferred to the household bathtub or shower. Its favorite dwelling place is between the fourth and fifth toes, because these two are closest together and, lacking ventilation, hold moisture longer.

Using a foot antiperspirant regularly will cut down on the moisture that makes you an easy target for fungi. The best I know of is an old country remedy, *powdered alum,* dusted lightly on the feet, between the toes, and in the shoes. As a disinfectant, use a light dusting of *powdered flowers of sulphur* in the same way. Regular use of *borated talcum* is a good preventive, and, in the early stages, it will often stop the fungoid growth before it starts to spread. There are several other antiperspirants on the market, but it's important to choose one that's mild enough not to irritate the tender skin that you're trying to protect.

Sheepherders have given the world a unique, homespun protection against athlete's foot: *small pieces of lamb's wool,* placed between the toes to absorb moisture. Dampened lightly with grated garlic or garlic juice, the lamb's wool, it is reported, can cure many cases that have started to spread. In the absence of lamb's wool, absorbent cotton will do, though it's not nearly as absorbent.

Giving the feet sun and air baths, ten to fifteen minutes a day, can produce excellent results. Air provides some of the ventilation they need, and sunshine, in moderate amounts, is both drying and healing.

Because fungi thrive best in an alkaline environment, and

foot-moisture is highly alkaline, it's a good idea to change your foot-environment to acid. Better than any costly drugstore medicine is this homemade antifungal preparation: *equal parts of cider vinegar and ethyl alcohol* sponged between the toes. Water may be substituted for the ethyl alcohol, to restore the skin's acid mantle, but it is not nearly as effective a fungicide as the vinegar-alcohol preparation.

Today, as always, every family can benefit by knowing when and how to use natural home remedies. But a word of caution: When a critical illness strikes or a serious injury occurs, there is no substitute for swift professional diagnosis and treatment. After the crisis has passed, home treatments can again be of great value in helping the patient to regain his strength, in keeping him comfortable, and in speeding his recovery.

Used regularly as preventive measures, some of the home remedies you've just read about can do such a good job of protecting your health that you can avoid much future illness. For many of these remedies, the cost is only pennies per treatment—sometimes even less.

So isn't it time you got acquainted with them?

RECIPES FOR MINOR
ACHES AND PAINS

**Boils
and
Infections**

Home Hypertonic Solution

1 pint hot water
1 teaspoon bicarbonate of soda
1 tablespoon Epsom salts
1 teaspoon boric acid

Mix all ingredients and stir until dissolved. Apply as a hot compress or use as a soak (but be sure it isn't hot enough to burn the skin). The same solution may be made with ice water and used as a cold compress or soak for acute inflammation, bruises, and swellings.

Poultices—American Indian

1. Raw carrot poultice: The original remedy consisted of shredded carrot mixed with a little wheat flour for a thicker consistency, but if I were using it, I'd substitute wheat germ—for the healing power of its vitamin E content.

2. Raw potato poultice: Wrap a scraped raw potato in a layer of cheesecloth and apply to the infected area. Or it may be thickened with wheat germ as above.

3. Roasted onion poultice: Cut the roasted onion in half and apply warm (but not hot enough to burn) to the boil. If you're hungry, you can eat the other half of the onion—if not, save it to reheat for a second application.

4. Lemon and fig poultice: A thick slice of lemon or a fig cut in half, heated and applied warm.

**Bruises
and
Contusions**

To Strengthen Capillaries and Prevent Bruising—From Germany

6 lemons
1½ quarts water

Wash and cut lemons, peel and all, in small pieces. Place in a saucepan, cover with water, and bring to a boil. Turn off the heat and let stand, covered, until cool. Pour into a jar with a tightly fitting cover and refrigerate. Let stand overnight before using.

Dosage: one cupful of the strained liquid two or three times a day.

Note: Lemons and all citrus fruits are rich in vitamin C, but it's the peel and the white skin under it that contain the bioflavonoids. Both are essential to strengthen the small capillaries, so give them a chance to work as a team.

Burns

Vitamin E-Herbal Burn Remedy—
From Germany

½ cup wheat germ oil (rich in vitamin E, it helps relieve
   pain, speed healing, and prevent scars)
½ cup honey (to heal and detoxify)
   comfrey leaves (to allay inflammation, promote healing,
   and aid the body in restoring damaged skin and
   tissues)

Place the wheat germ oil and honey in an electric blender
and let run at low speed until blended. Add enough comfrey
leaves to make a thick paste, and blend at medium speed to a
smooth mixture. Store in refrigerator to keep oil from becoming
rancid.

6

You Can't Cure a Cold, But . . .

Some years ago, my daughter was corresponding with a young draftee-boyfriend, stationed in one of the Army's northernmost outposts. His letters were filled with complaints about endless acres of snow, unyielding subzero temperature and constant bouts with running nose and sore throat. The pills prescribed by the medics afforded temporary relief, at best, and frequently left him with dryness, a wicked cough, and a mighty "hangover."

In one fell swoop, his disposition changed. It all began with a letter that read:

DEAR LORDEEN,

I've got a great new addition to your father's collection of folk remedies. It was taught to me by an Eskimo. He overheard me grousing, one morning, about my stuffed nose. Without a word, he picked up a handful of snow and told me to stick my nose into it. I thought he was putting me on, but he meant it.

"What the hell?" I figured. "Nothing else seems to work. Maybe these Eskimos know something we 'civilized' people don't." So I closed my eyes, took a deep breath, and plunged my nose into the wad of snow.

You know something? It worked! I mean, it really *works*—better than any pill! It clears out the nose in seconds, and it leaves no dryness, no coughing, no aftereffects whatsoever!

What a pleasure to be able to breathe again through my nose!

Fondly,
GREG

73

That was indeed a new and happy addition to my compilation of folk remedies, though it came as no surprise. For centuries, the residents of Iceland have treated a stuffed, swollen nose by immersing it repeatedly in a basin of cold water. Quite possibly, that's a variation of the snow treatment, taught by the Eskimos to the Nordic explorers who first touched their shores.

My daughter's young friend had simply discovered a fact long-recognized in the treatment of colds: *Heat expands, cold contracts.* By contracting the swollen membranes of his breathing passages, the freezing snow caused them to expel accumulated mucus. If Greg were aware of some findings about decongestants, antihistamines, and antibiotics, he would also have understood why that simple Eskimo treatment worked so much better than the medics' pills.

True, antihistamines have a temporary drying effect. But according to Dr. Richard B. Hornick of the University of Maryland School of Medicine, this drying effect "can backfire in a sense by precipitating an intractable cough due to the dry mucous membranes."

"Backfiring" is not the only danger in commercial cold remedies. Says Dr. Hornick, "Drugs used as nasal decongestants may indeed relieve a stuffy nose, but they may also interfere with the body's defense mechanisms against infection."

Another authority, Dr. Sol Katz of Georgetown University, is of the opinion that cold and cough medicines often have a "wild, irrational mixture of ingredients that can have harmful effects." Dr. Katz revived a famous old Jewish mothers' remedy, when he declared, "Hot chicken soup is very good. Hot drinks are good to break up a cold. They can make you feel much better than a lot of expensive cold remedies on the market."

As for antibiotics, once hailed as a veritable cure for the common cold, Dr. Henry E. Simmons described a survey in which he found that sixty percent of people with colds are given an antibiotic prescription by their doctors. Of all hospital patients who receive antibiotics, the survey showed, sixty percent of the cases do not need them. Dr. Simmons further warned: "The inappropriate use of an antibiotic can result in the appearance of resistant strains of bacteria with an increased number of superinfections each year, of which thirty to fifty percent are fatal."

A standard joke among doctors goes: "If I treat a patient for a common cold, he's usually over it in seven days. If he isn't treated, it hangs on for a week!" In other words, there is no known cure for the common cold.

The common cold is a virus infection, and the medical dictionaries give some important points to remember about virus diseases:

1. *Most drugs are ineffective against virus diseases.*
2. *Only the body can form substances which prevent the growth of the virus.*
3. *Virus diseases are usually highly infectious.*
4. *All viruses are destroyed by boiling.*

Doctors' prescriptions, as well as over-the-counter drugs, are frequently not only a waste of money but also a drain on the body's innate ability to combat the cold with built-in, natural defense mechanisms. You can help your body by following the basic laws for healthful living that build up your resistance to disease.

Sufficient rest and relaxation are important factors. So is physical activity, including some form of regular exercise suited to your age and way of life. But one of the best defenses against colds and illnesses was summed up in a single sentence by the author of a medical dictionary, Dr. Robert E. Rothenberg: *"A good state of nutrition should be maintained."*

Is there anybody today who doesn't know that the basis of good nutrition is a diet consisting of fresh fruit and vegetables, dairy products, whole grains, with special emphasis on the complete proteins of meat, fish, poultry, and eggs? Less well known is the fact that protein is used by the body to build antibodies. Without antibodies, your body would be unable to fight off the viruses that continually invade it.

Chances are, if you're a healthy individual, with no record of respiratory ailments, you can get away with ignoring a cold and letting it run its course. But why wait around for the virus to attack, when you can start a program for counterattack with your very next meal? Tests have shown that within a week on a high-protein diet, the body's production of antibodies can increase more than one hundred times, and, in many cases, a noticeable increase occurs within a matter of hours.

Giving your body the protein and vitamins it requires to

form the substances that stop the growth of a virus may be all the protection you need against colds. An overwhelming amount of evidence has shown that vitamin C, taken in large amounts, performs a variety of functions that make it one of the finest cold preventives and remedies available.

Like protein, vitamin C builds up the body's defenses by stimulating the production of antibodies. Its effects are almost miraculous in fighting infection and all types of viruses. It increases the bacteria-destroying ability of the white blood cells, and when a resistant strain of virus or bacteria isn't destroyed outright, its encounter with vitamin C inhibits its growth and makes it harmless.

Which is why, no doubt, the Indian tribes of Ecuador eat fresh, ripe acerola cherries as a cold preventive and fever remedy. Throughout much of South America, especially Ecuador, the acerola cherry grows in abundance. This particular strain of cherry is rich in vitamin C—so rich, in fact, that much of the acerola cherry crop is sold to American industries for use in many juices and foods, including some baby foods, to supplement their vitamin C content.

For colds, coughs, bronchial congestion, and asthmatic conditions, many of the Ecuadorian Indian tribes brew an infusion of acerola cherry stems. It's made by pouring two cups of boiling water over the stems, then covering and steeping for fifteen minutes. After it is strained, they add a half-cup of honey to make a syrup.

Though the Ecuadorian Indian tribes have scant knowledge of vitamin therapy, their treatment for colds tends to prove that even small amounts of vitamin C will provide some protection. Modern research indicates that the recommended dose, at the first symptoms of a cold, is from 1,000 to 3,000 milligrams a day. Doctors will tell you that there is no immunity against colds, yet all of them admit that some persons simply never have colds. I am one such person, and I think that I owe much of my immunity to the fact that, for years, I have taken three to six 500-milligram tablets of vitamin C daily.

Recently, a Hungarian scientist and Nobel Prize winner, Dr. Albert Szent-Györgyi, told of a combination of ingredients that his experiments had proved most effective in fighting the common cold. Dr. Szent-Györgyi—who with Dr. Linus Pauling, another Nobel laureate, is one of the great pioneers in vitamin C research—makes this recommendation: *In addition to 1,000 or more milligrams of vitamin C a day, add two ounces of wheat germ to the daily diet.*

That's because wheat germ is a good source of protein and the B vitamins, including the two best known for building up resistance to infection and stress: vitamin B_6 and pantothenic acid. Along with preventing colds, Dr. Szent-Györgyi's combination of nutrients also maintains a good state of general health.

To this advice, which I've dispensed often, I frequently get the reply, "Great, Lelord, but what if I already have a cold? What do I do for *immediate* relief of a stuffed nose, bleary eyes, sore throat, and coughing?" That's where the folk remedies can prove helpful—especially those that have been adopted by modern medicine.

Taking his lead from the Eskimo-Icelandic treatment for nose colds, one American physician put together a combination of ingredients available in most kitchens. It consists of two cups of ice-cold water, a teaspoonful of bicarbonate of soda, and a tablespoonful of Epsom salts.

After mixing the ingredients and stirring until thoroughly dissolved, dip a folded washcloth into the solution, squeeze out the excess water, and place it over the nose and sinuses. This process can be renewed as often as necessary to keep the compress cold enough to chill the nose, contract the swollen nasal passages, relieve the congestion, and lower the nasal temperature.

A more sophisticated variation of the ancient folk remedy was developed by two Israeli researchers, Dr. Menahem Ram of the Rothschild Hospital-Technion at Haifa, and Aladar Schwartz, an engineering researcher at the Israel Institute of Technology. After a long series of successful tests, these scientists believe they may have produced not merely a remedy but a cure.

In the Israeli hospital, the big toes of patients with colds were chilled with a refrigerant chemical. This treatment works, say Dr. Ram and Mr. Schwartz, because the big toes and the nose are nervous system reflectors of one another in their response to stress. A sudden, temporary chilling of the big toes promptly causes a lowering of the normal temperature within the nose. The combination of reducing nasal temperature and lowering the humidity results in a natural drying of the nostrils, a normalizing of the mucous membranes—and therefore, perhaps, a "cure."

A home variant of this treatment consists of dunking the toes in a basin of ice water containing floating ice cubes, and keeping the toes submerged until they're thoroughly chilled. Though ice water doesn't produce the same degree of chilling as a refrigerant chemical, it's been known to work almost as effectively.

The drying effect it produces is similar to the drying effect of antihistamines. However, the dryness from toe chilling is a natural, controlled process, not excessive enough to injure the mucous membranes. And there are no bad side effects—unless you consider two temporarily chilled, slightly numb toes as "bad side effects"!

What the trial-and-error methods of the ancient folk healers recognized was the need for moisture in the healing of nose colds. Under normal conditions, your inner nose lining spreads an invisible film of mucus that traps the germs you breathe. Dry, heated air can cause excessive dryness and cracking that break down this defense system. To build it up again, moisturization is necessary.

Most successful folk remedies are effective because they relieve dryness, prevent cracking, and help restore germ-proofing moisture to the nose. Like all treatments, they draw their ingredients from the vegetation native to their particular territories.

Thus, a New England remedy for nasal congestion and head colds is made by boiling equal parts of cider vinegar and water and inhaling the fumes. Natives of Formosa chip pieces of wood and bark from camphor trees, simmer them in boiling water, and inhale the fumes to clear the head and nasal passages. Or they make their own substitute for commercial camphorated oil by dissolving a half-ounce of camphor in two ounces of vegetable oil, and rubbing it around and under the nose. For a chest cold, they add a half-teaspoon of cayenne to the camphor-and-oil combination, mix it thoroughly, and rub it on the chest.

In Africa, a small pinch of cayenne pepper is sniffed to provoke sneezing and clear the nasal passages. To break up either a head or chest cold, a favorite African remedy is to simmer two teaspoonfuls of chopped fresh cayenne pepper and two tablespoonfuls of diced onion in a cup of boiling water for ten minutes. Strain and drink hot at bedtime or during the day as needed. If you don't have fresh pepper, try substituting a quarter-teaspoon of ground cayenne from your spice shelf.

On the tropical islands of Zanzibar and Pemba, the natives prepare a vaporizing solution and inhalant by putting two teaspoonfuls of cloves in a pint of boiling water; then they breathe in the fumes and moisture. The same inhalant makes a good substitute for tincture of benzoin in boiling water, long known as an effective home remedy for laryngitis. For chest colds, coughs, and bronchial disorders, inhaling the fumes and sipping clove tea (made by steeping four or five cloves in a cup of boiling water) provide triple benefits as an expectorant, a mild antiseptic, and a germicide.

In many parts of Asia, a vaporizing remedy, which is swallowed instead of inhaled, is said to be especially effective in treating sore throat and infected tonsils. A pint of milk and an ounce of chopped fresh ginger root are simmered in a small teakettle or heat-resistant teapot. The patient opens his mouth, holds it over the spout as close to the rising steam as he can without discomfort, and swallows the vapors. Two teaspoonfuls of powdered ginger may be used when no fresh root is available.

Another Asian remedy and cold preventive is to chew a small piece of fresh ginger root three times a day before meals. Or you can drink ginger tea; this is made by dissolving a quarter-teaspoonful of powdered ginger and two teaspoonfuls of honey in a cup of hot water. Ginger acts as an expectorant and helps relieve congestion in the bronchial tubes.

In the English countryside, a tea made of ginger and sweetened with honey is taken hot at bedtime, to break up a cold.

If you happen to keep a yak in your backyard, you might try this remedy from Outer Mongolia: To a cup of hot yak milk, add one teaspoonful of grated garlic and two tablespoonfuls of ghee. Drink it half an hour before bedtime, to break up a cold. Ghee is made by melting yak butter, cooling it, then pouring off the more liquid portion, which is the ghee. For those of you who don't keep yaks around the house, you can make your ghee the way the East Indians do—from the butter of buffalo milk!

For colds, however, the Indians prefer a fruit remedy that's long been used in warm climates as a cooling drink, a mild laxative, and a fever breaker. It is, to quote a Colonial physician, "a substance of great use in both putrid and inflammatory disorders, for abating colds, fever, and thirst, and keeping the belly soluble."

This versatile Indian remedy is made by pouring a quart of boiling water over one cup of tamarind pulp, which is then covered and infused for two hours. After straining the infusion, a teaspoonful of honey is added to a half-cup of the liquid, then diluted with water to suit the taste. It is taken every three to four hours, and the best results are achieved when it's sipped slowly.

"Eat the pomegranate," Muhammad advised his disciples, "for it purges the system of hatred and envy." Today, Muhammad might be disenchanted with its effect on hatred and envy, but pomegranate is still used beneficially, in Arabia, for a variety of ailments that include canker sores, sore throat, colds, fever, and coughs.

To make a gargle, simmer two tablespoonfuls of dried pomegranate rind in three cups of water for twenty minutes. Cool, strain, and use undiluted for an irritated throat and cold or for canker sores. (Unlike tamarind, fresh pomegranates are available in American markets during the season.)

An Arabian friend tells me that there is no over-the-counter product in our country or abroad that reduces fever as effectively —or as safely—as pomegranate juice. Getting the juice from a pomegranate could be a tedious job unless you have a juicer, so my suggestion would be to eat the fruit very slowly, letting the juice trickle down the throat. Or you can purchase bottled pomegranate juice at all health-food stores.

In Finland, fresh lingonberries are simmered, pureed, and mixed with honey for a cold and cough remedy so delicious that you'll enjoy taking it even after you're well. And those who never have colds can get its many nutritive benefits by eating it for dessert. Canned lingonberries, as well as the juice, may be substituted if the fresh fruit is not available.

In the United States, England, Scotland, and other parts of Europe, where black currants are obtainable, they may be substituted for lingonberries, with maybe better results. Black currants have long been used as an ingredient in cough syrups and lozenges. Glycerine and black currant pastilles are an old-time favorite that's still popular, especially in England.

Another Central and South American remedy—for head colds, running noses, fever, and a host of other ailments—consists of a strong tea made of sarsaparilla root. Make the tea by using one ounce of sarsaparilla root to each pint of water and simmering the mixture for thirty minutes. Drink a small cupful three or four times a day and at bedtime. For extra benefits and flavor, sweeten it with honey and add a squeeze of lemon.

The Chinese, in the past twenty years, have emerged from centuries of ignorance and superstition. But even as their scientists learn the most modern techniques of healing, they continue to separate fact from superstition. The result has been a blending of modern science with the wisdom of the ancients. From their vast, age-old storehouse of folk medicines come a number of cold remedies that are still in use today.

Chu chi is the Chinese term for lard. Mixed with roasted onions, the lard is rubbed on the chest to loosen deep-seated coughs.

Hsia ku ts'ao is a blue-flowered Eurasian herb of the mint family. It's been naturalized throughout North America, and generations of Chinese have found that it lives up to its English name of *self-heal.* They consider *hot self-heal tea,* made from one ounce of the plant to one pint of boiling water, a valuable aid in relieving the discomforts of a cold and in speeding the patient's recovery.

T'ien men tung is a vegetable that has many medicinal properties. In China, it's made into a soup or puree and served hot, as a cold remedy and "to soften dry coughs." In America, many of us are aware of its health benefits, but we eat it because we enjoy it. It's known as *asparagus!*

Gypsy cold and cough remedies usually consist of herbs and fruits in season, in various combinations with bark, roots, seeds, honey, lemon, and other simple ingredients that can be obtained wherever the gypsies travel. Angelica and nettle tea are the easiest to prepare, since all you need are tea bags from your health-food store and boiling water. Gypsies usually pick and dry their own herbs, and, whenever possible, they add those two universal cold remedies, honey and lemon. They have found that a good hot brew of herb tea, with honey and lemon, not only helps relieve the symptoms of a cold, but aids in cold prevention. And if they're out of tea, they substitute a popular American remedy, hot lemonade and honey.

Other herb teas favored by gypsies as cold remedies are avens, comfrey, coltsfoot, black cohosh, and hyssop.

A famous gypsy remedy for cough or chest cold consists of a decoction made by boiling nettle leaves, licorice root, and enough honey to make a syrup.

In France a delicious cough remedy is made by stewing ripe, red cherries in just enough water to cover, with honey added to make a syrupy consistency. Cool, remove the cherry pits, and add lemon juice to taste. Take it by the tablespoonful—if you can resist gobbling it all up for dessert!

With an unlikely combination of ingredients, the Scotch and Irish make an easily prepared and inexpensive cough remedy. Scrub but do not peel a large white turnip. Slice off the bottom so it will have a flat bottom to stand on. Cut in half and divide each half into three or four slices. Cover each slice with honey and place the slices together again in a small bowl to form a whole turnip. Drizzle two tablespoonfuls of honey over the turnip, and let stand for four hours, or overnight if possible. By that time the turnip juice and honey will have combined to form a syrup that Irish friends tell me "never fails to stop a cough before it gets a grip on you and goes into grippe."

Buy your turnips with the tops on and cook the greens for the fringe benefits of their high vitamin and mineral content. And don't throw out the water they're cooked in: A cup of the hot "pot likker" contains valuable nutrients and can help to break up a cold. If that isn't inducement enough to cook the greens, there's an old Irish saying that contains more truth than blarney: "Eat turnip tops and grow beautiful!"

In Greece, a delicious, demulcent cough remedy is made by stewing figs, honey, and lemon slices to a soft consistency. Take a tablespoonful as needed or whenever you like.

An old German remedy for colds and flu is a tea that you can enjoy whether you're sick or well. It's made by pouring boiling water over equal parts of peppermint and elder flowers, one teaspoonful of each (or a tea bag of each) to one and a half cups of water. Steep five minutes, strain, and drink while hot. As a cough remedy, reduce the amount of water to half a cup, add three tablespoonfuls of honey and the juice of half a lemon.

I don't know who gave the herb called pleurisy root its name, but long before it had a name the Natchez Indians drank a tea made by boiling the roots, to cure pleurisy, coughs, bronchitis, and other respiratory complaints, including pneumonia.

Creosote bush, also known as greasewood, is a native of the Western states, and was used for numerous ailments by Indian tribes of the Southwest. Long before creosote was official in the United States *Pharmacopoeia,* as an expectorant and pulmonary antiseptic, Indians were drinking a decoction of the leaves for chest colds and other conditions, and using it as a gargle or chewing the leaves as an expectorant.

When molasses became available to the Indians, the Mohegans made a cough syrup by simmering mullein leaves in equal amounts of water and molasses.

The Ojibwas, Mohegans, and Potawatomis used the inner bark of white pine to make a tea for coughs and colds. The Objibwas also concocted a cold remedy from the bark of wild cherry trees, and made a cooling beverage for colds and fever by boiling the cherries, squeezing the juice and diluting with water.

The bark of white pine and wild cherry were both listed later in the United States *Pharmacopoeia* and used in commercial remedies for colds and coughs.

To cure a head cold and to stop running noses, the Potawatomis dried the roots of sweet flag, reduced it to a powder, and sniffed it. Other Indian tribes chewed the roots as a cold remedy, or made a tea by simmering the roots in water.

COLD PREVENTIVES TO WEAR
AROUND YOUR NECK

These alleged cold preventives, once very popular, are now seldom heard of except in a few rural areas. There's only one reason why they may have some merit; see if you can figure it out.

From Russia: a dried herring wrapped in a cloth, tied with a string.

From Italy: a small bag filled with garlic cloves.

From Australia: a bag of camphor.

Even from the United States: Americans bypassed all the other odorous remedies in favor of one that smelled even worse. Young old-timers can still remember the asafetida bags they used to wear to school, especially in rural districts.

Have you guessed the reason why all these "preventives" might work? Obviously, because they smell so bad! Since nobody will come near you, there's less chance of exposure to colds and flu!

As I write this, a really effective preventive of the common cold has been tested successfully on volunteers by a Stanford University scientist and a British medical research team.

"This is the first agent known to prevent common cold infections in man," said Dr. Thomas C. Merigan, chief of the Division of Infectious Diseases at Stanford University, and his collaborators from the Common Cold Unit at Harvard Hospital in Salisbury, England.

The remedy they used is interferon, a protein produced by the body in response to a virus attack. But there's a catch to it, as the scientists were careful to point out: There is no way yet to manufacture interferon in mass production, and an effective dose at present costs several thousand dollars.

Until mass production brings the price of interferon down low enough for everyone to afford it, your best preventive is to keep up your body's natural defenses by maintaining a good state of nutrition and adding plenty of vitamin C and wheat germ to your daily diet.

Meanwhile, if you do feel a cold coming on, remember that all of the tested remedies—even some that sounded the strangest—have proved beneficial in treating one or more of the symptoms. Though you can't expect them to cure a cold that already has a head start, years of home treatment and recent modern experiments have shown that most of these remedies can relieve many of the discomforts of a cold and, in the majority of cases, help you get well faster.

Best of all, these mixtures contain no antibiotics, membrane-drying antihistamines, or resistance-lowering decongestants.

COLD REMEDIES FROM
AROUND THE WORLD

Asia
Minor

Spice and Honey Plaster

2 ounces powdered ginger
1 ounce powdered cinnamon
½ ounce powdered mustard
2 teaspoons red pepper
honey

Mix the dry ingredients with enough honey to form a smooth consistency. Spread on a cloth (preferably flannel or flannelette) and apply to the chest, leaving it on overnight.

Omit the honey and mix the spices with pure lard or vaseline and you'll have an ointment to rub on the congested area.

England

Ginger-Citrus Cold Remedy

6 lemons
4 oranges
¼ pound seedless raisins
3 cups honey
3 ounces ginger root (macerated)
1 gallon water

Wash the lemons and oranges and squeeze the juice from them. Refrigerate juice to use later. Add all the other ingredients to the water in a large saucepan, bring to a boil and simmer for an hour. Skim off the top when necessary. Remove from the fire, pour into a large pitcher or jar and leave overnight. Add lemon and orange juice the next day. Drink two or three cups a day.

To make ginger wine, stir in ¼ oz of yeast when the juice is added. Stir every day for ten days. Strain, pour into a small cask or stone crock, but don't close until all fermentation is over. Cork tightly. Drink one wineglassful in a cup of hot water, preferably at bedtime.

Poland

Remedy to Break Up a Cold

1 cup milk
1 tablespoon honey
1 teaspoon butter
½ teaspoon grated fresh garlic

Heat milk until it's scalding hot. Add honey and butter and stir until honey and butter are well mixed. Add garlic. Garlic powder can be used as a substitute if no fresh garlic bulbs are available. Drink slowly about an hour before retiring.

Canada

Moisturizing Nose Spray

2 cups water
1 teaspoon salt
2 tablespoons glycerine

Mix ingredients and stir until the salt is dissolved. Pour into a sterilized bottle or jar with a lid. To use, fill a small atomizer with the solution and spray the nose with it two or three times a day, or as needed.

Iceland

Remedy to Break Up a Cold

1 tablespoon chopped onion
1 cup barley water
2 teaspoons cod-liver oil

Simmer the chopped onion in the barley water for ten minutes. Remove from the fire, add the cod-liver oil, stir and drink while hot. May be taken as needed during the day and preferably at bedtime.

Two teaspoonfuls of safflower oil or one teaspoonful of butter may be substituted for the cod-liver oil. One half cup of barley water with a teaspoonful of salt and a tablespoonful of vinegar makes an excellent gargle.

Russia

Herbal-Licorice Decoction

1 tablespoon plantain leaves
1 tablespoon coltsfoot leaves
3 cups water
½ ounce licorice root

Place herbs and licorice root in a scalded teapot or jar with a cover. Boil the water and pour it over the herbs. Cover and steep for twenty minutes. Strain. Take a small cupful, hot, three or four times a day.

Russian Herbal-Pine Remedy

1 quart water
1 ounce marshmallow root
¼ ounce pine needles
½ ounce each of dried mullein flowers, sage leaves, and anise seed

Place all herbs and dry ingredients in a scalded teapot or jar with a cover. Boil the water and pour it over ingredients. Cover and steep for twenty minutes. Strain. Take one half cupful (preferably hot) three times a day and before retiring. (Most of these herbs are available in health-food stores among herb teas.)

Russian Herbal Gargle

1 tablespoon linden tea (or tea bag)
1 tablespoon sage tea (or tea bag)
1 tablespoon camomile tea (or tea bag)
1 ounce oak bark (if available)

Pour one and a half pints of boiling water over them and steep, covered, for thirty minutes. Use as a gargle as often as needed for throat irritation and inflammation and as a refreshing mouthwash.

Gypsy

Romany Herbal-Ginger Remedy

1 ounce white horehound
1 ounce hyssop
2 ounces coltsfoot
1 ounce lump ginger
2 quarts water

Simmer all ingredients in boiling water until the liquid is reduced to one quart. Cool and strain.

Gypsy Cough and Chest Cold Remedy

2 tablespoons whole linseeds
1 quart water
2 lemons
½ cup honey

Simmer linseeds in water for an hour and fifteen minutes. Strain. Squeeze lemons and add the juice and the honey.

7

Fruits: The Remedies That Revitalize

The medical world called him a quack, but that didn't stop droves of heart-attack sufferers from beating a path to his door. His name was Dr. Green, and his office, located in Ennis, Ireland, had become the last refuge of patients throughout the British Isles—victims of coronary thrombosis, angina pectoris, myocardial degeneration, and other fancy-named afflictions. Many were invalids, close to death.

Statistics are sparse for that period—the late nineteenth century—but if reports of his own patients bear any validity, Dr. Green's treatment was truly astonishing. People to whom mere walking was an effort could now go through a normal day's activity without the slightest loss of breath. In many cases, palpitations and chest pains were reduced to a minimum. Edema, the painful bloating of bodily cavities, was frequently reduced or eliminated, as long as the patients maintained the therapy.

Unfortunately, the good doctor was a bit of a showman and opportunist. He refused to divulge the "secret" of his treatment —another reason, no doubt, why he was labeled a charlatan. Upon his death, in 1894, his niece finally revealed the mysterious remedy. It turned out to be a tincture derived from the plant *Crataegus oxyacantha*, popularly known as the hawthorn berry.

To herbalists and naturopaths, there was nothing surprising about this revelation. Back in the seventeenth century, Nicholas Culpeper wrote of the hawthorn berry: "The seeds, beaten to powder being drank in wine, are held singularly good against the stone, and are good for the dropsy (edema). The seed cleared from the down, bruised, boiled in wine and drank, is good for inward tormenting pain." Though somewhat exagerated, these claims later led to widespread use of the hawthorn berry as a tonic, especially in the treatment of cardiac asthma, edema, and sclerosis (hardening of the arteries).

What Culpeper, and those who followed him, never knew was that the hawthorn berry had the same uses, among American Indians, for ages. Tribes of the northwest gave it the names of *ashnum asho* and *we nap ish*. They ate it lavishly, to guard against heart attack.

Histories of fruits abound with folklore and romance. Like all remedies of bygone ages, the discovery of their curative properties came by accident, and their uses were confined to the areas in which they grew abundantly. Not until the Age of Exploration did their fame spread. Many fruits, which we now take for granted as kitchen staples, have long medical backgrounds.

When Captain Cook embarked on his voyages, in the sixteenth century, British seamen were plagued by scurvy, a disease that caused swelling and bleeding of the gums, livid spots on the skin, and extreme exhaustion. Arriving in the South Pacific, Cook was fascinated by the complete absence of this dread disease among the native islanders. He also observed that they consumed great quantities of lemon.

At once, the captain ordered his crews placed on a daily lemon-ration. To a man, the symptoms vanished rapidly, and scurvy was literally wiped out. In all parts of the world where citrus fruits—lemons, limes, oranges, grapefruit—are eaten, scurvy does not occur.

Science later learned the reason: vitamin C. This potent nutrient not only cures scurvy, but is effective against a long list of everyday ailments, including the common cold. Tahitian natives relieve a sore throat by gargling with pure lemon juice. Tribesmen of the Solomon Islands treat symptoms of asthma by drinking large quantities of the juice. Among the American Indians, fever is treated by the Florida Seminoles with massive doses of orange and grapefruit juice.

Because they are rich in vital minerals—calcium, magnesium, phosphorus, potassium, and sulfur—citrus fruits form the basis of many folk remedies. Indonesian natives chew on whole lemons, rind and all, to ward off the ravages of rheumatism. Since Biblical times, Palestinians have valued the laxative effects of an orange-rind decoction, because it stimulates the tissues of the bowel. Gout sufferers, on the island of Pago Pago, eat every part of the lemon except the rind, which they then apply as a poultice over the painful joint. The Seminoles chew grapefruit seeds vigorously, then swallow them, as a cure for worms.

Since Elizabethan times, English farmers have used orange and lemon rinds to loosen corns and to remove warts. For treating teen-agers with acne and blackheads, the farmers rub lemon juice directly onto the skin and leave it to dry. This treatment also bleaches out freckles.

Where citrus fruits were once scarce, another fruit rich in vitamin C, the cherry, performed many of the same medicinal functions. Japanese peasants downed cherries by the bucketful, to relieve the pain of arthritis and gout. For bronchial and asthmatic attacks, they prepared a decoction from cherry stems, which was then strained, cooled, and turned into a syrup with honey. From this homemade medicine, they also derived the benefits of malic acid, a fever reducer and diuretic (kidney stimulant).

Another fruit with the same health-giving nutrients is the apple. Also rich in pectin, an ingredient used widely in commercial binding medicines, apples are a worldwide folk remedy for diarrhea. Russian peasants treat the condition by simmering pared apple in boiled milk, drinking a warm half cupful every hour until relief comes. Silesian farmers believe that only the top part of the apple cures diarrhea, while the bottom part is effective against constipation.

Apples yield another foodstuff that has proven of great medicinal value: cider. In Normandy, France, where unsweetened cider is drunk as a beverage, kidney stones are virtually unknown, while gout and rheumatism hardly touch the peasant population. These facts are attributed to the diuretic action of the concentrated malic acid, which eliminates poisonous uric acid from the body. The slight acidity of cider also destroys putrefactive bacteria associated with gout.

In many parts of England, Scotland, and Germany, apple

cider vinegar is used as a lotion to shrink varicose veins. The country folk of Vermont apply this lotion as a remedy for shingles, night sweats, burns, impetigo, and ringworm. Mixed with an equal part of water, it speeds the healing of poison ivy rash. Combined with egg yolk and turpentine, it relieves lameness.

Rare indeed is the fruit that doesn't contain some medicinal properties. If you have any favorites, which you eat regularly, chances are you're protecting yourself against a number of afflictions. Fruits are most effective in their natural states, unmarred by chemical fertilizers and insecticides. Most canned fruits and fruit juices lose their nutritional and medicinal value in the processing plants. Too often they're packed in heavily sugared syrup, which counteracts the beneficial effects. Artificial preservatives may keep them on the market shelves longer, but those same preservatives can damage your health.

Canned or frozen strawberries, for example, taste great, but their food value leaves much to be desired. In their natural state, however, strawberries, in the words of Culpeper, are "singularly good for the healing of many ills." Culpeper was seconded by the great Swedish biologist, Linnaeus, whose experiments showed strawberries to be a virtual cure for gout and rheumatism.

American Indians treated numerous stomach ailments with a tea brewed from strawberry roots. Strawberry preserves are an ancient Indian delicacy. Swedish farmers consider the strawberry better than any toothpaste: To prevent tartar, they cut the fruit in half and rub the juice over their teeth. The Swedes also eat strawberries to eliminate kidney stones and skin disorders. Because strawberries, too, contain vitamin C, citric and malic acids —plus a number of trace minerals—herbalists since ancient times have regarded them as a blood-purifier.

Growing wild, the entire berry family has a unique talent: It's likely to pop up anywhere. Any forest is loaded with berry bushes of all varieties. They are not uncommon in parks and sometimes appear even in vacant lots.

Gathering berries is a romantic old custom. Gathering medicine—that's something else! And yet, whenever you go picking berries, that's just what you're doing! Did you know, for example, that the common blackberry plant has been used, since

Biblical times, as a cure for dysentery? Mixed with honey, a decoction of the unripe roots and berries is a favored sore throat remedy among the Malays of Indonesia. And bartenders, who claim to be "authorities" on any subject, are quick to prescribe a famous old folk remedy for diarrhea: blackberry brandy or cordial.

Cranberries, less widespread than blackberries, grow abundantly in the bogs of Cape Cod, Massachusetts. In a sense, they were once a godsend, because the cranberry, rich in ascorbic acid, became a staple on every whaling vessel. Like citrus fruits, it prevented scurvy among the crews.

The Pequot Indians, who once inhabited that territory, brewed thick cranberry drinks as medicines for fever and asthmatic attacks, while the Wampanoags made poultices of crushed cranberries, to remove boils and fever blisters. Among the old families of Cape Cod, housewives still serve lightly cooked cranberries as a remedy for high blood pressure, poor complexion, and skin eruptions. New England herbalists are very high on cranberries as a blood purifier—eaten without sugar, of course.

Long before the discovery of insulin, many folk cultures were using one of nature's remedies for diabetes: the blueberry. Later, research showed that blueberry leaves are rich in *myrtillin*, a substance that dissolves blood sugar. On the island of Crete, many natives still prefer the cure for diabetes handed down by their ancestors: a teaspoonful of dried, cut blueberry leaves, steeped in a cup of hot water, and taken every six hours. The berries themselves, rich in minerals, are eaten by these people to purify the blood. Infusions from the roots and stems are drunk as medicine for kidney troubles.

Black currants, the raisinlike berries that grow profusely in The Levant, are a basic ingredient of many commercial gargles, cough syrups, and lozenges. But Lebanese women still prefer to boil black currants into a syrup for inflamed throats and bronchitis, while Syrian farmers prepare an infusion from the young roots, for sore throat and fever.

Raspberries, which grow in a variety of colors, were long ago used by Algonquin medicine men to cure scrofula, the tuberculous disease that causes swelling and degeneration of the lymph glands. In recent times, European doctors have been treating the same condition with large doses of pure raspberry juice. The red raspberry is still used extensively in childbirth.

Among the Macedonians of Yugoslavia, expectant mothers are encouraged to drink strong infusions of red raspberry leaves and roots, to ease labor pains and reduce the risk of miscarriage. Macedonian women also drink a decoction of the same ingredients, to ease the pain of menstruation. English farmers use a similar infusion to remedy diarrhea, and they chew raw raspberries to keep their teeth clean.

When vintners turned the elderberry into one of the world's favorite wines, could they have foreseen its value as medicine, too? English farmers make a thick syrup out of elderberries and comfrey decoction, to relieve bronchial complaints. Elderberries, whether drunk as wine or tea, induce heavy perspiration; this makes them a worldwide remedy for fever.

Berber tribesmen, in the northwest plains of Morocco, have adapted the gooseberry as a remedy for many ills. Mashed together with figs, gooseberries become the ingredient of a gentle but efficient laxative and worm expellent. When Berber men and women advance in years, they nibble on gooseberries to ward off arthritis and liver complaints. A strong, bitter brew of the leaves and stems is said to dissolve gallstones.

Throughout the northern hemisphere, there grows a genus of trees that are put to many uses. The wood of one variety is used to build chests and closets. Another member of this genus yields a flavoring used in gin, and still another gives an oil used in medicines and perfumes. Collectively, these trees are called junipers, and their berries provide one of the oldest folk remedies known to man.

All five tribes of the Iroquois Confederacy ate chopped juniper berries to heal urinary disorders. A strong berry infusion was used as a lotion for snakebites and the stings of bees or poisonous insects. Berry tea was a cure for colicky infants and a general remedy for cramps.

The Burgots of Mongolia consider a juniper root and leaf decoction a potent relaxant; they feed it to pregnant women when labor starts. A much stronger, thicker decoction, brewed from the stems, is a Burgot remedy for piles and bleeding gums. Burgots nibble on the berries when they need to expel excess gas.

Long before the cause of diabetes was known, the Lillooets of Canada brewed their own native remedy: huckleberry leaf tea. This ancient tribe cultivated huckleberries for many other ailments, as well. Crushed and spread over animal skins, the raw berries were applied as poultices for serious cuts and bruises. Root decoctions were fed to tribesmen suffering from high blood pressure, and leaf teas were drunk to cure looseness of the bowels. Tribal law required that an overweight Lillooet go on a strict fast, eating nothing but huckleberries.

The mulberry, another fruit common to northern climes, has an ancient history in Chinese folk medicine. Oriental healers prescribed a leaf decoction for constipation and a root infusion for diarrhea. Chewed plain, the berries were considered an excellent relief for liver troubles. Mashed berries were spread on the skin for such diverse conditions as acne, ringworm, impetigo, and hives.

Unlike berries, many fruits are still waiting to be "discovered" by the average housewife. This is a pity because some have long medical histories, confirmed under the rigorous scrutiny of modern science. Probably the best example is the papaya.

When Hernando Cortez led his conquering army through Mexico during the sixteenth century, they arrived in Yucatán, the land inhabited by the ancient Mayas. There, according to the journal of Cortez's chaplain, the soldiers were wined and dined by the Maya chieftains—fed all manner of native dishes that left them bloated from indigestion.

At last came the dessert—a sliced golden melon which the Spaniards had never seen before. Already stuffed to the gills, they sampled the strange new fruit with mixed feelings of fear and curiosity. Within a few swallows, their attitude turned to amazement—for the sweet, thirst-quenching melon had completely relieved their stomach distress!

Ababai was what the Mayas called this marvelous fruit. The Spanish translated the word into "papaya." Its fame spread rapidly, as Cortez planted it on Mexico's western coast, where Captain Cook later discovered it and carried it across the Pacific. Eventually, it wound up growing in just about every tropical clime.

Native inhabitants were no less amazed than Cortez's warriors, and numerous folklores grew up around the papaya. Still prevalent is the belief that the papaya tree is part human, because it produces male and female flowers on separate plants, and the fruit takes nine months to develop. Because of its unique benefits, many tribes still call it the medicine tree.

Wherever the papaya tree grows, natives tenderize their meats by wrapping them in the green leaves or by rubbing them with the juice of the unripe fruit. And, like the Mayas, they eat the unripe fruit to curb indigestion. These two seemingly unrelated "talents" of papaya flow from its main ingredient, papain, which exists nowhere else in nature.

Papain is an enzyme that breaks down protein foods to a digestible state. Applied to meat, it penetrates the tough fiber and gristle, rendering them soft and chewable. If you keep commercial meat tenderizer in your pantry, read the contents on the package. You'll notice that its chief ingredient is papain, obtained from the papaya.

In your stomach, papain performs the same function. For unlike the other enzymes found in foods, and the juices your stomach walls secrete, papain works in any kind of medium—acid, alkaline or neutral. And while most enzymes confine their action to specific types of food, papain works on all types—protein, fats, and carbohydrates.

So you may well ask, if papain breaks down any food it comes in contact with, what about the tissues of your digestive tract? Built of the same elements as the meats we eat, wouldn't they be affected, too? Therein lies the answer to the papaya's fabulous feats as a food and medicine.

For some reason still not clear, papain is a very selective enzyme: *It only breaks down food and dead tissue.* Thus, as a cure for simple indigestion or chronic dyspepsia, the value of papaya is obvious. But its medicinal uses go further, much further.

Apply its milky juice to boils and contusions—as the Dayaks of Indonesia do—and it promotes healing by destroying scar tissue, without damaging healthy skin. The Dayaks also use papaya juice to dissolve corns, warts, and pimples. In Seminole country, where papaya trees now grow, the Indians treat ulcerated skin and open wounds by wrapping them in fresh papaya leaves.

Centuries before modern science brought immunization and vaccination to primitive peoples, they were beating papaya pulp into a paste, which dissolved the false membrane of diphtheria. They devoured large quantities of the fruit to heal ulcers and other forms of internal bleeding. Many brewed the leaves into mild decoctions or strong infusions, to remedy constipation or diarrhea.

The Bahutus of Africa make a papaya paste to destroy ringworms. For internal worms, they chew and swallow the seeds of the papaya. The Batwa pygmies, when struck by sore, inflamed, or infected gums, soak them in a mouthful of juice. This not only heals the tissues but also dissolves pus. Throughout all of Africa and South Asia, native tribes use papaya juice to dissolve the discharge of ear infections.

Indians and Pakistanis eat extra papaya when troubled by piles, enlarged liver, or spleen. To relieve pain in nursing mothers, they roast lightly bruised papaya leaves and apply them to the breasts. Women all over the tropics rub papaya juice on their faces, to remove freckles and other blemishes. By destroying only dead cells, the juice also "tenderizes" the skin into a soft, smooth consistency.

While modern medicine has already begun to make use of powdered papaya and papain extract, the fruit's greatest potential is yet to be realized. Records of the ancient Incas show that their medicine men performed complicated surgery, and used papaya to heal incisions. Inca lore also tells how papaya dissolved tumors and arrested the spread of malignancies.

Sheer legend? Tall tales of tribal storytellers? Maybe. But in light of papaya's proven properties, science is not yet ready to laugh them off.

Because papaya is highly perishable, the melon is difficult to ship much beyond its native habitat. Until this transportation problem is solved, the papaya is not likely to become a household fruit outside the tropics. In the meantime you can enjoy a more common tropical fruit that offers many of the same values: the pineapple.

Fresh pineapple is still a popular cure for dyspepsia and indigestion among natives of the Hawaiian Islands. It contains an enzyme called bromelin, which has the same protein-digesting traits as papain. Also harmless to healthy tissue, pure pineapple juice is a native remedy for sore, inflamed throats. In such widely separated lands as India and Brazil, pineapple juice is an ancient remedy for intestinal worms.

Though papaya seems to be a more potent medicine, pineapple has one advantage over its tropical cousin. By the time papaya is fully ripened, most of the papain has been neutralized, rendered useless. Not so for the bromelin in pineapple, which maintains its strength even when the fruit is completely ripe. Remember, though, that only the *fresh* pineapple contains medicinal value. Once subjected to the canning process, the whole fruit or the juice are nothing more than refreshments.

Few fruits contain the all-encompassing medicinal value of the papaya, but practically every one has something to offer in the way of folk remedies. Like all medicinal foods, they possess distinct advantages over drugs. They never become habit forming. They cause no harmful side effects, except to the allergic or those who gorge themselves. At the same time as they alleviate ailments, they provide the body with nutrition.

Dates, for instance, are rich in vitamins and minerals. Boiled in water, they produce a sweet liquid that Arabs have used for centuries as a laxative. Arab physicians also prescribed dates for nervousness, piles, and poor circulation. Figs, too, are an ancient Middle Eastern remedy for constipation.

While jouncing on the hump of a camel, many years ago, I discovered still another use for figs. One of my traveling companions developed a severely inflamed boil that was causing him no end of pain. As he bemoaned his fate, hundreds of miles from the nearest doctor, our Arab guide halted the caravan and withdrew a large fig from his food sack. Splitting open the fruit, he immersed it for a few minutes in warm water. He then mashed the softened fig onto a gauze bandage, which he taped onto my friend's boil. Within a few hours, the boil was gone!

"Where did you learn that treatment?" I asked the caravan guide.

"From your Old Testament," he replied. "It is written in Isaiah that Hezekiah, the King of Judah, used this same treatment to cure boils."

I subsequently discovered that Arabs also drink fig juice to heal sore throats and to ease indigestion. Externally, they apply fig poultices to relieve congestion of colds.

"Eat the pomegranate," wrote Muhammad, "for it purges the

system of hatred and envy." The full meaning of the great prophet's words have been lost in antiquity, but they symbolize the great respect accorded this native fruit. It was—and still is— used by Arabs to expel tapeworms, to heal sore throats, and to dissolve cankers of the mouth and throat. It also reduces fever, and its seeds are cooked to produce a syrup that heals inflamed mucous membrane.

The tamarind was another fruit prescribed by Arab physicians, since Biblical times, to reduce fever. Growing throughout the tropics, it is consumed as a laxative and diuretic by such diverse tribes as the Luo of Kenya, the Alfuro of Indonesia, and the Hova of Madagascar.

In the heart of equatorial Africa, bananas have been a traditional tribal medicine and strength-builder. Because this versatile fruit provides fast energy, natives carry it along on the hunt and other rigorous journeys. Its inner skin, applied as a poultice, speeds the healing of burns, wounds, and boils. The seeds, ground to a fine powder, are taken as a laxative. Mashed and mixed with boiled milk, bananas—skin and all—become a native remedy for diarrhea, colitis, and ulcers. Combined with honey, mashed bananas are used as a salve in the treatment of piles.

Where the equator cuts through Asia, another native fruit, the mango, is esteemed as a cure for numerous ills. Sulawesi inhabitants of Indonesia drain the mango's juice and drink it for all respiratory disorders. Ground into pulp, the fruit is rubbed over the body to tone up the skin and unclog the pores. In the Molucca Islands, natives mix mangoes with local herbs, then brew them into a decoction for kidney ailments and fever.

Guava, a berrylike fruit of equatorial America, is a native staple of that locale. Indians of Colombia drink the juice as a remedy for dyspepsia, and they chew on the stems when they sense rising blood pressure. In the Galápagos Islands, natives chop up and brew the entire plant into a syrupy decoction that is fed to asthma sufferers. Women of the Galápagos use tepid guava tea as a douche for excessive menstruation. Between menstrual periods, as a preventive, they eat a mixture of guava and ground coconuts.

Of course, it isn't necessary to travel halfway around the world to find native fruit remedies. Many exist in America's own backyard, so to speak.

Quince trees and shrubs, growing in various parts of the country, yield a fruit that was once used by Indians to heal sore mouth and throat and to soothe stomach upset. An infusion, brewed from the seeds, is an old Pilgrim remedy for patients convalescing from feverish colds. Pilgrims also considered this infusion the safest drops for sore eyes.

An infusion of the persimmon, which grows both in Asia and North America, has been used as a folk remedy for diarrhea and dysentery. The Algonquins brewed it as a gargle for sore throats. If "coffee nerves" are your problem, you might try an old Southland substitute: persimmon seeds—dried, roasted, and ground.

Need I mention prunes, one of the world's oldest laxative fruits? The only thing to remember is that prunes must be eaten raw if they're to work effectively. If they're too hard and dry for you in their natural state, don't cook them! Soaking them in cold water will render them just as tasty.

If you don't enjoy the taste of prunes, try them in their original state—as plums. Grown since pre-Biblical times in Asia, the plum is a relative newcomer to North America. In India, plums were eaten to relieve rheumatism and halt the spread of tumors. The Tamils of Ceylon still drink a plum-brew to relieve dyspepsia, bronchitis, and rheumatism. Wherever the plum grows, its laxative properties are lauded.

Another widely used laxative fruit is the pear. Ancient Chinese medicine also recognized pears' diuretic properties and prescribed ground pears in tea for kidney ailments. The Lusitanians of Portugal regard pears as a potent remedy for colitis and high blood pressure.

Tea, brewed from watermelon seeds, was a medicine for many Indian tribes, especially in the South. Yazoo witch-doctors administered it for heart attacks. Medicine men of the Koasati used it to reduce the swelling of edema. All of the Tonkawan tribes drank watermelon-seed tea to relieve high blood pressure. Creeks, Apalachees and Quapaws were among the many Indians who swallowed a strong infusion to expel worms.

Recent research explains why these watermelon cures must have worked. The seeds contain *cucurbocitrin,* a substance that dilates the capillaries, thus reducing pressure on the larger blood vessels. Another seed substance, tested in laboratories, was shown to paralyze tapeworms and roundworms in cats. Watermelon, which works to flush the kidneys, is an age-old preventive of two kidney diseases, nephrosis and nephritis.

Indian *shamans* also valued the peach tree. From the leaves, the Hitchitis brewed an infusion that was tranquilizing, slightly laxative, and an excellent remedy for morning sickness in pregnancy. Turning it into a syrup, they used it to clear congested passages and irritated membranes. The Appalachees made a leaf decoction that healed infected ears.

Reduced to a powder, peach leaves and bark were a universal Indian medicine for malaria, long before the discovery of quinine. When Guale tribesmen went on the warpath, they carried stores of powdered bark to rub on wounds. Santee medicine men had no idea of the iron contained in peaches, but they did know that the fruit, in large doses, could purify and strengthen the "tired blood" of their aged.

The apricot, rich in iron and vitamins, was another Indian blood strengthener. Women of the Miwok tribe, in California, fed their children a root-stem decoction for anemia, while elderly members of the tribe drank a steady diet of leaf tea. Asthmatic Miwoks relieved chronic spasms by inhaling the fumes of chopped, simmering apricots. Considered a bowel-cleanser, the fruits were eaten in large doses to relieve both constipation and diarrhea.

Slowly but surely, science is learning the reasons for the success of fruit remedies. One finding, of course, is the vast vitamin and mineral content of fruits. More intriguing is the germicidal nature of fruits. Each step forward, in the laboratories, brings further evidence that fruits—especially their seeds—contain true antibiotic substances. But there are many mysteries about fruit cures yet to be solved.

In this respect, grapes are perhaps the most fascinating of all fruits. Wherever they grow, grapes have been used to remedy a long list of ailments. But grapes have a very independent personality, because they do their best work only when the body is free of all other foods.

Centuries of experimentation, by remote native tribes and flourishing civilizations, eventually culminated in a cure that is now widespread—the grape-fast. Basically, this treatment consists of placing the patient on a rigid fast, allowing him only water for days, weeks, sometimes even months. He is then fed nothing but grapes, as often as ten times a day, until the illness abates.

There is little danger to the health in this treatment because grapes are loaded with nutrition. When Mahatma Gandhi went on his marathon fasts, for example, he sustained himself by drinking pure grape juice. But why are grapes, as medicine, practically useless if combined with other foods?

No one knows for sure. One theory holds that even the minutest amount of "alien" food dilutes the grape's potency by changing its chemical structure. It is also thought that grapes, which ferment rapidly, impart their fermentation to the other foods, releasing alcohol and poisons into the bloodstream. When eaten alone, grapes are digested before they have a chance to ferment.

Whatever the reason, European clinics have had remarkable success with the grape-fast. For people whose gums are swollen and teeth loosened by pyorrhea, the chewing of grapes, seeds and all, drains off the pus and strengthens the gum tissue around the teeth. In combination with fresh air and sunlight, it has brought tuberculosis patients back to health. Grape-fasts have been credited with curing pneumonia, arresting arthritis or rheumatism, and repairing damaged heart tissue. It is even claimed, by victims of terminal cancer, that the grape's powerful acids dissolved their malignancies!

Once a patient is pronounced cured, he's brought back, by stages, to normal eating. The grapes are first combined with other fruits, later with green vegetables and whole grains, and finally with lean red meats. Patients are urged to continue on a maintenance quota of grapes, fast occasionally for a day or two, and avoid the empty calories of sweets and refined carbohydrate foods.

Fruit fasting, in general, is an old folk remedy. In some tribes, like the Quechuas of Bolivia, a number of fruits are combined into a single cure. Other peoples go the route of the Burmese Chins, who have individual fruit fasts for different ailments.

Fasting, it should be cautioned, is not a frivolous matter. In the area of folk medicine, we moderns are strictly laymen. An occasional fast can't hurt—it may even be beneficial to general health—but a fast-cure should never be attempted without the advice and consent of a doctor.

Fruits are a powerhouse of energy. Eaten abundantly, they provide the body with vitamins and minerals that build up its natural resistance to disease. The curative properties in their stems, roots, leaves, and bark are transmitted in some measure to the fruit itself.

Whole fruits provide much greater benefits than the juice alone. However, if juice is your strict preference, at least be sure that it is fresh and unadulterated. Juice that stands for any length of time loses most of its nutritional and medicinal value.

The fruit kingdom may not be the answer to all of mankind's ills, but, as our forefathers proved, it goes a long way toward keeping us healthy. At the same time, fruits are fun to eat because they provide taste-tempting flavor and refreshment. What other medicine can make this boast?

FRUIT RECIPES FROM AROUND THE WORLD

Blood Purifier

Blueberry Blood Purifier—From Crete

Mix equal amounts of blueberries, thyme, watercress, and sassafras bark. Steep a teaspoonful of the mixture in a cup of hot water. Cover and let cool, then strain.

Dose: One cupful four times a day. Don't eat much food.

Digestion

Fruit Soup—From Switzerland

> 2 cups raisins
> 2 cups prunes
> 4 quarts cold water
> 1 cup unsweetened grape juice
> 2 lemons (peeled and sliced)
> honey

Soak raisins and prunes overnight in the water, then simmer until cooked. Add grape juice and lemons. Sweeten with honey to taste.

Diarrhea and Dysentery

Blackberry Remedy—From the Oneida Indians

> 1 ounce or 2 tablespoons blackberry roots
> 1½ pints water

Grind roots until they are very fine. Place in boiling water. Keep boiling until mixture is down to a pint.

Dose: One or two ounces, three or four times a day as necessary.

Blackberry Cordial*

* I recommend this only for people who feel they *must* taste sugar and alcohol in their medicine.

> 1 cup ripe blackberries
> 2 cups sugar, raw, unrefined
> 2 or 3 cloves
> 2 small pieces of cinnamon
> 1 pint hot water
>   port wine

Boil fruit, sugar, cloves, and cinnamon in water for ten minutes. Cool and strain. Add equal amount of port wine to the strained liquid.

Dose: One tablespoon in warm water as needed.

Fever

Tamarind—From the West Indies

> 1 ounce tamarind pulp
> 1 quart water

Steep pulp in boiling water for one hour. Strain when cool.

Dose: A half cup diluted with a little water every two or three hours.

Laxative

Tamarind—From the West Indies

> 1½ ounces tamarind pulp
> 1 ounce honey
> 1 ounce raspberries or strawberries

Mix ingredients well.

Dose: Two teaspoonfuls morning and night.

Compound of Figs—From Kuwait

2 ounces figs
2 ounces raisins
2 ounces barley
½ ounce licorice root
2 pints hot water

Boil figs, raisins, and barley in hot water for fifteen minutes. Add licorice root and allow it to soak into mixture. Let cool, stir and strain.

Dose: A half cupful night and morning.

Sore Throat, Throat Irritation and Sore Gums

Black Currant Cough Syrup—From Syria

2 heaping teaspoons black currants
2 cups hot water
1 tablespoon honey or raw brown sugar

Simmer—but do not boil—currants in hot water for ten minutes. Strain through cotton. Add honey or raw brown sugar to a cupful of the mixture while it is warm.

Dose: As often as required.

A Lebanese variation of this remedy omits the honey or raw brown sugar to turn it into a gargle.

Black Currant Gargle—From Israel

2 heaping teaspoons fresh black currants
(or 1 teaspoon dried)
1 glass hot water
½ teaspoon ground cinnamon

Simmer fruit in hot water for ten minutes. Add cinnamon and let mixture stand covered for one half hour. Strain and use warm.

Fig Gargle—From Egypt

½ ounce figs
½ ounce mallow root
1 pint milk

Cut figs and mallow root into small pieces and add to boiling milk. Simmer to three-quarters of the original amount.
Dose: As needed.

Pomegranate Gargle—From Syria

2 ounces or 2 tablespoons dried pomegranate rind
1½ pints hot water

Boil pomegranate rind in hot water until down to one pint. Strain and cool.
Dose: Undiluted as a gargle or applied to sore or bleeding gums.

Whooping Cough

Lemon Syrup—From England

1 lemon sliced thin
½ pint flaxseed
2 ounces honey
1 quart water

Simmer all ingredients in water for four hours. Do not boil. Cool and strain. Add enough water to make a pint if mixture has simmered down.
Dose: One tablespoon four times a day and an additional dose after a severe fit of coughing.

8

Natural Tranquilizers and Aids to Sleep

"You poor thing," my wife said, "you must have been frightened out of your wits."

"No" came the answer. "I was sleeping so soundly, I didn't hear a thing. In fact, I wasn't aware of *anything* happening till I woke up this morning."

And that's when my ears perked. We were talking to our friend Hal Peterson, whose home had just been stripped bare by burglars during the night. Closets were ransacked, bureau drawers lay strewn over the floors, even Hal's vault, containing his most valuable papers, had been wrenched open.

"It doesn't seem possible, Hal," I said. "Only last week you were complaining how lightly you sleep. You were having a real bout with insomnia."

"Not anymore," Hal said, "not since my doctor prescribed those marvelous sleeping pills. Now I sleep like a log."

It's a story I've heard often—and so have you. Sometimes the outcome is a lot more tragic. Like when people die in a fire because they were sleeping so soundly that they couldn't awaken in time. Or when lives are lost because someone was so fast asleep that he couldn't hear the ringing of an emergency phone call or a cry for help in the night.

More often than not, it's later discovered that the heavy sleepers were unable to awake because they were under the influence of sedatives or barbiturates—or both. Were they really "sleeping" or would it take some other term to describe their drug-induced state? To learn the answer, let's see what modern research has uncovered about the nature of sleep.

In experiments pioneered at the University of Chicago, numerous sleep laboratories around the country have been able to chart the behavior of the human body as it goes into sleep. By means of electrodes strapped to key points on the sleeper's body, an electroencephalograph (EEG) in an adjoining room records the minutest bodily changes. On moving strips of graph paper, pens automatically record variations in his rate of breathing, his heartbeat and pulsebeat, blood pressure, body temperature, muscle tone, eye movements, and, most important of all, the minutest variations in the voltage of his brain waves.

Employing volunteer subjects, researchers are also able to chart their sleep behavior under the influence of alcohol or drugs, certain foods, and sudden noise, light, or temperature changes. Sometimes a sleeper is abruptly awakened to find out if he was dreaming, and if he remembers the dream. Some of the subjects first spend twenty-four, forty-eight, even seventy-two hours of enforced wakefulness before going to sleep, to determine if that amount of strain makes a difference in their sleep patterns. The EEG also measures the behavior of volunteer insomniacs and all manner of "light" and "heavy" sleepers.

From studies of thousands of case histories, experimenters have come up with a portrait of an ideal night's sleep. Normal, healthy sleep takes place in four stages:

Stage I: After a moment in which you relax and your thoughts start to wander—usually with the eyes closed—you are awakened for a split second by a sudden jerk of the body, a tiny burst of activity, and then hurled into this opening stage of sleep. Your muscles relax further, your pulse starts to grow even, breathing becomes more regular, and your temperature begins to fall. If you were connected to an EEG, your brain waves would appear small, pinched, irregular, undergoing rapid changes. You are still aware of idle thoughts and dreams, maybe even a floating sensation, and if someone were to awaken you in this stage, you would likely maintain that you hadn't yet fallen asleep.

Stage II: As you descend to this next level of sleep, your eyes roll slowly from side to side, as your thoughts become fragmented and you begin to dream somewhat. Your eyes may still be open, but they see nothing. A small noise or light could awaken you, and you might still wonder if you'd been asleep at all. Your brain is still active, but the brain waves are swiftly growing larger.

Stage III: You have now been sleeping for about ten minutes, as your muscles move toward complete relaxation, your breathing grows even, and your heartbeat starts to slow down. Your temperature continues downward, blood pressure starts to drop, and it would take a quite loud noise to awaken you. The EEG traces slow, large brain waves at the rate of about one per second, indicating that the voltage from your brain is much higher, and changes are occurring more slowly.

Stage IV: Soon you enter this deepest stage of sleep. Dreams cease, unless you are prone to occasional nightmares, and you are most difficult to awaken. Breathing, heart rate and blood pressure continue even, and your temperature continues to fall. If you are a bed wetter or a sleepwalker, these problems occur during Stage IV. Researchers have named this the Delta Stage, because the brain-wave patterns—large, slow, and jagged—assume the triangular shape of the Greek letter *delta.*

REM: Stage IV is what people once considered the most beneficial form of sleep. The longer it lasted, the more physically sound and mentally alert you'd be during your waking hours. In the normal healthy human, modern sleep laboratories have proven otherwise. For within twenty minutes of entering this stage, you start to drift back upward, your sleep growing lighter and lighter, to a point of near-wakefulness. Though it is difficult to awaken you, your brain waves become small and irregular, as if you *were* awakening. Your fingers and toes twitch, while your blood pressure, pulse, and breathing become irregular. Most significant of all, you start to dream vividly, and you seem to be watching those dreams as you would watch TV or a movie—with rapid eye movements (REM). It is now some seventy to ninety minutes since you first fell asleep.

The first REM period lasts about ten minutes, and then the sleeper descends again for another sojourn in Stage IV. Soon he is drifting upward to another REM session, and then back downward. This cycle occurs four to five times during the night, but as morning approaches, the sleeper doesn't sink to the very bottom of Stage IV, his stay there is briefer, and the moment of REM lasts longer.

As the body prepares to awaken, brain waves start to resume their daytime pattern, as do the heartbeat, pulse, respiration rate and blood pressure. Upon awakening, you may recall a fraction of your REM dreams, or you may not remember dreaming at all: Actually, most of your sleep was accompanied by dreams.

I spelled out this sleep pattern in some detail because it helps to shed some light on the hazards of factory-made drugs as compared to the natural remedies for insomnia. Drugs, while seeming to induce deep sleep, tend to distort the normal four-stage pattern. Subsequent experiments in sleep laboratories have indicated that it is unhealthy, even dangerous, to keep a person too long in the depths of Delta Sleep.

Stage IV is certainly the most restful sleep period, and if it's lengthened by natural means, the results can be beneficial, particularly to the person who has trouble falling asleep. But the most desirable, healthful night's sleep is one that includes the frequent trips up to REM.

Though unfamiliar with the four stages and REM, the Kurds of Iraq long ago recognized this fact. According to their ancient, religious traditions, a sleeper cannot awaken fully rested, with a clear head, unless he rids his brain of stored-up dreams. To this end, the Kurds drink curdled (no pun intended!) goat's milk from a goatskin bag. The bag is then placed under the head, and the sleeper positions his face toward Mecca. Deep sleep, filled with dreams, follows swiftly.

Goat's milk is also an insomnia remedy for the mountain folk of Greece. Heated, then mixed with a tablespoon of honey and liberally sprinkled with nutmeg, it is drunk as a nightcap.

Milk as a sleep inducer is native to many cultures, but only recently have experiments demonstrated why. One of the amino acids in milk, tryptophane, was fed to volunteers in an experiment at the University of Oklahoma. All the subjects fell asleep more quickly, awakened less often, and derived longer benefits from Stage IV. Some moved more rapidly up to the REM period, but all of them awakened feeling well rested and refreshed.

Compare this reaction to a typical drug-induced sleep. The user drops into a deep torpor, frequently without passing through the normal stages. He rarely experiences REM until the latter part of the morning, when the drug's effects start to wear off. At that point, the body starts to make up for lost REM time, causing intense, long-lasting dreams that chemically excite the brain. The drugged sleeper, upon awakening, then wonders why he still feels groggy and irritable, even though the pill gave him a "good night's sleep."

In its soured, acidulated forms—buttermilk, yogurt, sour cream, etc.—milk is a source of calcium, another nutrient associated with sleep. Which is why the long-lived Abkhasians and the hardy Balkan mountaineers down an extra tumbler or two of buttermilk at bedtime, when troubled with restlessness. They not only achieve healthy, uninterrupted sleep, but their bodies derive a "bonus" in the form of lactic acid and other ingredients that promote all-around health.

How does this dual advantage stack up against the use of sleeping pills? Increased drug consumption in the United States has been accompanied by a rise in *iatrogenic illnesses*—conditions caused by the use of drugs. Many sleeping tablets contain aminopyrine, or Pyramidon, both of which destroy the white corpuscles in some people's blood. When this happens, resistance to infection drops so low that a common cold may result in sudden death. More than 1,300 recent deaths in this country have been attributed to the use of sedatives which contain these drugs.

Blood and liver diseases have been shown, in many cases, to be induced by the excessive use of tranquilizers, as has Parkinson's disease, an affliction characterized by uncontrollable tics and tremors. Barbiturates, over a long stretch of time, can cause irreparable brain damage.

Like the Kurds, Burmese natives also attach a religious mystique to sleep. They believe that restlessness is dangerous during the night, because the sleeper may awaken while his soul is still out wandering. So, at the first sign of sleep difficulty, a Burmese takes massive nightly doses of plant pollen—in the form of pollen-cakes and loose powder. This treatment may continue for weeks, even months, until the user is assured of uninterrupted slumber. When treatment ceases, there are no ill aftereffects, no harsh withdrawal symptoms—and the cure is lasting.

Once again, a comparison. Sedatives and barbiturates—even many of the "mild" over-the-counter tranquilizers—have one result in common: dependency. With steady use, the insomniac soon discovers that he can't possibly fall asleep without them—

in bigger and bigger doses. Veteran pill-poppers take as many as fifty to sixty pills a day because they not only need them to sleep but they also need them to satisfy a physical craving. Once a person is habituated or addicted, the devastating side effects drive them to their doctors or hospitals for a cure.

And that's when withdrawal symptoms begin, even when the patient is taken off the drug gradually. Frightening hallucinations or convulsions, similar to epileptic seizures, are not uncommon. Extreme depression frequently sets in, sometimes resulting in a suicidal urge. Memory becomes faulty, often to the point of complete amnesia. The mind loses much of its reasoning capacity, as simple jobs—like adding numbers, writing sentences—become a superstrain on the brain. Fever, dehydration, and rapid weight loss may occur, resulting, finally, in heart failure.

Are sleeping pills worth all these risks? It would hardly seem so in the face of the ultimate outcome of withdrawal. Even if withdrawal symptoms are mild, insomnia swiftly returns, worse than ever, leaving the patient right back where he started!

There are no dependency or withdrawal symptoms in a remedy handed down by the cave-dwelling Pueblo Indians. It consists of large doses of mushrooms at bedtime. Mushrooms are rich in the B vitamins, which are also considered a factor in healthy sleep.

An ancient Chinese extract would hardly be classified as a drug. It is made from equal parts of dried orange peel and ginseng, fortified with honey. Taken just before going to bed, it produces sleep that is both restful and revitalizing.

The natives of the West Indies make use of a beautiful indigenous vine to calm the nerves and promote sleep. It is called *Passiflora* (passion flower) and here is what one authority, Dr. Swinburne Clymer, tells us about it:

"It is an antispasmodic and mild soporific [sleep inducer]. It is indicated in asthenic [weakening] insomnia and also in the restlessness and insomnia of low fevers. *Passiflora* should be given in all feverish conditions where there is extreme nervousness and lack of sleep. It is quieting and soothing to the nervous system. *Passiflora takes the place of narcotics.*"

An old English farmers' remedy for insomnia is a tea made by simmering three or four chopped lettuce leaves in a cup and a half of water. After twenty minutes the tea is strained and taken as a bedtime beverage.

Irish country dwellers prepare the same mixture and add sprigs of fresh mint. If it's a stomachache that's keeping you awake, the mint helps relieve that condition, too.

An old Scandinavian folk remedy is to soak a pad of cotton wool in cider vinegar. You must hold it close to the nose and inhale deeply, until the nostrils begin to prickle. Then lie perfectly still—unless you can't keep from scratching your nose!

In the Scottish countryside, oatmeal gruel is used not only as a builder-upper but also as a go-to-sleeper. Just cook oatmeal in the usual way, but with enough water to make the gruel thin. Sweeten with honey and drink at bedtime.

Until recently, the nature of sleep and insomnia were too often misconstrued. Sleep laboratories have cast a whole new light on some old wives' tales.

For one thing, there is no "proper" amount of sleep that is the same for every individual. Nor is there a "best time" for sleeping. My grandmother, an excellent sleeper, believed avidly in the dictum laid down nearly two thousand years ago by the great Hebrew scholar, Maimonides: "The day and night is twenty-four hours. It is enough for a man to sleep one-third of them." Grandma also believed that the best sleep occurs before midnight.

Both these rules have been proven erroneous. The quantity of sleep a person needs depends on his build, his weight, and on the amount of physical and mental activity he performs in the course of a day. People who take catnaps require less sleep at night. Sedentary workers need less sleep than those who perform heavy manual labor, although people who engage in prolonged, intensive mental activity often need the most sleep of all.

As for *when* the best sleep occurs, there is no special time. Your deepest and longest descent into Stage IV takes place at the beginning of sleep, no matter what time you turn in, day or night. For example, Eskimos of the Far North, where "day" and "night" last approximately six months, have no concept for a "proper time" for sleep.

Perhaps more than any other peoples, Eskimos rely on the biological "human time clock" to tell them when they must sleep. But in order to assure that all members of a tribe will sleep at the same time, a restless Eskimo brings on sleep by swallowing powdered animal bones. That's not so wild when you realize that bones are loaded with sleep-inducing calcium.

Individual calcium foods are the bases of numerous folk remedies for insomnia. Tribes of the outlying Hawaiian Islands rely on large night-time doses of ground coconut meat. In the soul food sections of the South, extra quantities of raw okra are said to induce a healthy drowsiness. Bedouin Arabs resort to the soporific effects of figs.

A number of herb teas are centuries-old remedies for tension and insomnia. They are: anise seed, bergamot, birch leaf, chamomile, catnip, dandelion, hops, lobelia, rosemary, and valerian. Gelsemium, also known as yellow jasmine or wild woodbine, adds extra relaxing benefits to the nerves in the arterial blood vessels.

Like sleep, the condition known as insomnia also defies guidelines. Few people can lie in bed for an entire night without achieving some amount of sleep. Many so-called insomniacs find that they sleep well for a few hours, awaken rested for a couple hours more, then grow sleepy again as dawn approaches. Under the omnipresent sensors of the sleep laboratories, most "light sleepers" are surprised to discover that they actually sleep soundly for hours on end, without realizing it. Except for people with certain rare illnesses or damage to the nervous system, there is no such thing as *total* insomnia.

But, of course, the world we live in demands that we adhere to some sort of sleep regime—one that allows us to face the waking hours refreshed and to go through the day free of drowsiness, tension, and irritability. A period of wakefulness, which is calm and tranquil, helps to overcome the vicious circle brought on by a night of troubled sleep. A "bad" day programs the mind and body for a "bad" night—and vice versa.

Many of the folk remedies that I described as soporifics are also excellent as tranquilizers during the waking hours, when taken in smaller quantities. There are also tranquilizing activities that require no food at all.

The yogis of India, famous for their relaxing exercises and bodily contortions, have handed down a "tranquilizer" that requires no training or practice. Called a *yoga slant board,* it consists simply of a board elevated twelve to fifteen inches at the foot-end. After strapping the feet, to prevent slipping, you lie in that elevated position for about fifteen minutes. The resulting flow of blood toward the brain is said to produce a feeling of well-being far superior to any drug *or* food.

Among the Hindus, the slant board is a standard piece of furniture in the home and at the place of work. They resort to it frequently throughout the day and at bedtime. If you're the athletic type, you can achieve the same results through another yoga method—standing on your head from three to five minutes!

The Tosk peoples of southern Albania believe that mental tension is caused by physical tension in different parts of the body. Using the sense of touch, they seek out these tense spots, which usually turn up in the neck, the shoulders, or the small of the back. They then apply moist heat, in the form of a compress, until the tightness vanishes—and with it, the "tightness" of the brain.

To achieve both daytime relaxation and a good night's sleep, the Sephardic Jews of the Middle East simply apply warm compresses to their eyes. This natural tranquilizer was handed down by their ancestors, the Talmudic scholars, who spent long hours reading and interpreting the Hebraic laws, much to the strain of their eyes.

In Persia the tribes people still practice a simple technique taught to their ancestors by the wise men of Babylon. It consists of inhaling deep breaths through the mouth and exhaling through the nose. They continue breathing in this manner until overcome by a feeling of relaxation and well-being. Further continuation lulls them into a sound sleep.

The Tigreans of Ethiopia achieve the same results by simply yawning themselves into a state of relaxation or sleep. They do this by opening their mouths as wide as possible, straining and stretching the muscles of the jaws and neck. At the same time, they breathe in and out as deeply as possible, until a gradual state of relaxation sets in. At that point they return to their day's labors or turn over and go to sleep.

If you own a compass, you might like to try an ancient yoga technique, which Charles Dickens adhered to faithfully. After determining the direction of true north, turn your bed so that the head faces in this direction. Why? Because, according to yoga theory, magnetic currents flow north and south between the poles, and you will sleep much better if those currents pass in a straight line through your body!

Or "When you are waked up by uneasiness and find you cannot sleep easily again, get out of bed, beat up and turn your pillow, shake the bedclothes well with at least twenty shakes, then throw the bed open and leave it to cool." This was the advice of Ben Franklin, which went on, "In the meanwhile, continuing undressed, walk about your chamber, till your skin has had time to discharge its load, which it will do sooner, as the air may be drier and colder. When you begin to feel the cold air unpleasant, then return to your bed. You will soon fall asleep, and your sleep will be sweet and pleasant."

If you're the adventuresome type, you might try stuffing your pillows with hops, as many troubled sleepers in England do. Scotch and Irish country folk have handed down a "lullaby" pillow stuffed with a combination of hops and catnip or mugwort and rosemary. The mugwort, it is alleged, promotes pleasant dreams, while the rosemary keeps away evil spirits!

Instead of popping tranquilizers for relaxation, you can just as easily carry around tranquilizing snacks that have stood the test of time. Many Chinese calm their nerves with soybeans or rice polishings. Greek peasants munch on carob. An old American farmers' remedy is to down a mouthful of bran flakes. All of these foods contain one or more of the nutrients conducive to relaxation or sound sleep.

Of course, no amount of sleep aids can work to perfection unless the *conditions* for sleep are right. By eliminating outside glares and noises, you can overcome two major sources of sleep disturbance. A sturdy mattress, free of lumps and hollows, which "gives" according to the shape of your body, further enhances restful sleep. A pillow that doesn't twist your head way out of line is also helpful. So, too, is a single fluffy blanket, compared to the weight of numerous thin blankets.

And, finally, the greatest natural aids of all: a proper diet and a positive state of mind. Caffeine, alcohol, and other stimulants are definitely taboo for insomniacs. A well-rounded food program containing the B vitamins, calcium, lactic acid—foods that "feed" the sleep center of the brain—is the best route to sound sleep and relaxed wakefulness. If, however, your brain insists on remaining active, and no amount of natural sleep aids seem to help, don't go near those pills! You're better off getting out of bed to read or to watch the TV late show, until drowsiness finally overcomes you. Whatever sleep you lost can be recaptured on the following night.

It is important for you to remember, in training your mind, that sleep is a time for escape and forgetfulness. This is what my grandmother must have meant when she taught me her own special rhyme:

> *The problems you face in the day ahead*
> *Will never be solved by worry in bed!*

9

Remedies the Gypsies Taught Me

"Tell me, little one, what is it that grows head down and feet up?"

"I don't know, Taras. Tell me."

"An onion, little one! And did you know that if you eat an onion at bedtime, you will sleep like the wintering bear?"

I was six years old then, spending my first summer at my Uncle Casimir's farm. Taras was a *lafkye*—a traveling Gypsy. Each year he and his *malkóch*—his tribe—made camp on the outskirts of my uncle's pastures, where they tilled the soil and performed odd jobs for the local populace. At the end of fall harvesting, they folded their *katúnas*—tents—and set out for warmer climes.

Uncle Casimir had a special affinity for Gypsies, perhaps because he'd grown up among them in the old country. No more "tolerated" in America than they were in their native lands, Gypsies could always feel welcome in this little oasis of hospitality.

As for myself, it was my first experience with Gypsies. Unlike the stereotypes that had already formed in my mind, Taras and his people were not fortune-tellers, con men, or thieves. With each succeeding summer, I came away from the farm a little older and a lot wiser, thanks to the earthy wisdom they imparted to me.

Having lived off *poshik*—the soil—for centuries, Gypsies were (and probably still are) the world's foremost authorities on natural healing. Gypsy medicine *is* folk medicine, handed down from generation to generation by word of mouth. Their favorite way of teaching was to begin each "lesson" with a riddle—and Taras was no exception.

"Little one," he asked me that same summer, "what grows in a garden yet never turns green?"

I felt sure he was trying to trick me, and I wasn't about to take the bait. "Aw, come on, Taras! There's a little green in everything that grows."

"Everything, little one? Even mushrooms?"

I'd been "had" again! But Taras didn't stop there. He rarely did. As I said, his riddles were frequently a takeoff to some knowledge he was about to impart.

Gypsies eat lots of mushrooms, he told me, because mushrooms grow everywhere. "They bring strength to the blood and beauty to the skin," he explained. At the first sign of acne, eczema, whiteheads, and other similar conditions, Gypsies down large quantities of mushrooms.

"Do you know why our eyes never burn?" Taras went on. "Why our lips and tongues never grow sores? Why our hair and skin are never too oily? Because we eat mushrooms in great number."

Years later I was to learn that mushrooms are a good source of riboflavin and niacin. Without realizing it, Taras was "prescribing" two nutrients that are necessary to maintain healthy skin and blood! He also taught me a Gypsy secret for keeping mushrooms potent right up to the moment of eating: Never peel them. To clean them, simply rub the skin with a bit of salt.

Not all foods are so easily available as mushrooms. As wanderers, Gypsies have had to live off whatever vegetation was available in a particular locale. By no means are they confirmed vegetarians, but most Gypsies I've met, starting with Taras, because of economics, eat *mang* (meat) sparingly. But they make sure their diet has an adequate supply of herbs, nuts, and vegetables. *Anros* (eggs) and *chuti* (milk) are dietary staples, considered powerful preventives against childhood illnesses. And while you'd never catch a Gypsy buying *jumeri* (bread) in a store, they eat large quantities of home-baked breads made only with whole grains.

Gypsies had not only a great talent for discovery, but also a great willingness to learn. Wherever they halted their *vardos* (caravans), even if only for a few hours, they swiftly absorbed the local folklore, including folk medicines. With an instinct for experiment, they then combined what they learned with what they already knew, producing countless concoctions for whatever might ail the human body.

Till this very day, *lafkyes* have no respect for orthodox medicine. They consider the druggist *drabengro*—maker of poison. Any doctor is *mulled-moosh-engro*—maker of dead men!

Many of the Gypsies' cures, as Taras taught me over the years, are as close as the nearest kitchen or garden. A true Gypsy, however, will never go to the kitchen if the garden is within reach because he believes that the medicine is strongest when plucked from the soil.

For all manner of skin diseases, Gypsies eat grated raw potato. They also nibble on raw potato simply to maintain the health of the hair and skin. Celery juice is another ancient Gypsy remedy for blemished skin. Stewed celery, served in its own juice, is eaten by Gypsies to reduce high blood pressure and to ease the pain of rheumatism. These conditions are also treated with an infusion brewed from the seeds. Rheumatism and high blood pressure can also be checked, according to the Gypsies, by drinking cucumber juice. Skin conditions are also relieved by drinking spinach juice and carrot juice.

When blood pressure falls too low, Gypsies drink large quantities of beet-root juice, which they also regard as a blood builder. Tomato juice is said to purify the blood, and prune juice acts as a blood tonic.

"If you wish to remain *shastó*—healthy—little one," said Taras over and over again, "drink of the fruits that cleanse *rati*—the blood." This was almost a religious belief among the Gypsies. In each *katuna* on my uncle's farm, no family was ever without a crock filled with at least one of the blood-purifying juices.

When more than one was available, they were combined. The women's favorite recipe consisted of chopped carrot, celery, and spinach, mixed in equal amounts. After adding chopped parsley, they simmered the mixture in a small quantity of water until every bit of juice was extracted.

Many herbs, which today are used to season and flavor foods, were considered far more valuable by the Gypsies. For nervousness or upset stomach, they added greater amounts of marjoram to their dishes. Kidney trouble and poor appetite were treated with chives. Cloves, caraway seeds, and cayenne pepper were aids to digestion.

Thyme played a very important role in Gypsy medicine. Brewed into a tea, it was taken to relieve coughs, colds, and asthmatic complaints. When available, flaxseed and honey were added, to strengthen and soothe. Thyme tea was drunk to relieve headaches and to induce restful sleep.

Horseradish was also high on the list of Gypsy remedies. To relieve the pain of neuralgia, they held a small bag of freshly scraped horseradish root to the pained area. Mixed with a little water, the ground roots turned into a deep-heating compress for the relief of tension, stiffness, and pain in the back of the neck.

Because of its antiseptic properties, Gypsies take horseradish for coughs, colds, and bronchitis, and they eat the leaves of the plant to combat food poisoning. They add horseradish to vegetable juices to stimulate digestion and to aid the passing of urine through faulty kidneys. For rheumatic pains, they either eat the horseradish or mix it with boiled milk as a compress. Other conditions treated with horseradish are asthma, dropsy, catarrh, low blood pressure, poor appetite, and poor complexion.

The horseradish-milk concoction is also used as a cure for freckles. Applied cold to the freckled skin area, it is left to dry for a half hour, then removed with tepid water. This treatment is repeated every two or three days until the freckles vanish.

Their unique life-style naturally led Gypsies to create remedies that made living more comfortable. Being wanderers, they instinctively searched for ways to strengthen the feet and legs.

"In our feet lies the secret of our survival," said Taras. "When a *lafkye* loses his power to walk, he loses his wish for life."

Small wonder that Taras and his tribesmen—and Gypsies the world over—never wore shoes unless absolutely necessary. From infancy, they learned to walk barefooted. This, explained Taras, toughened the bones of the feet and made the skin thick and horny.

Gypsies go out of their way to walk in dewy grass because they believe that this further toughens the soles. For the same reason, wading through salt water is an ancient Gypsy foot-builder. When they anticipate a long journey, they rub their feet with a brew of pounded-up ivy leaves that have soaked in warm vinegar for two days.

There are times, of course, when even a Gypsy must trudge with covered feet. To prevent tiredness and heat buildup, he'll line his boots or socks with cabbage or mallow leaves. If these are not available, he'll dust his toes with cold wood ash, finely burned, or cold smoked-out tobacco ash.

"And now, little one, tell me what it is that fills the eyes before it feeds the belly."

By now I was a few summers older, but that one had me stumped.

"Mustard!" Taras responded to my blank, helpless gaze. "I speak not of the mustard that your mama buys in the *fóros*—the marketplace—but of the plant that grows to a height of three feet, its leaves burning with the fire of the devil."

I was already aware that Gypsies used the chopped leaves and seeds of the mustard plant in great abundance, not only to pickle and flavor their foods but also to aid digestion. What Taras taught me was the unique medicinal uses that Gypsies made of mustard.

An ancient Gypsy remedy for constipation is to nibble on fresh mustard leaves while cooling the mouth and throat with sips of water. If a Gypsy needs to induce vomiting, he brews a seed decoction (about one teaspoonful to a cup of water), waits till it's lukewarm, then downs it in one gulp. For simple digestive distress, Gypsies drink a mild, tepid infusion made from the leaves.

Gypsies rarely suffer from head or lung congestion. On the rare occasions when they do, they steep ground mustard seeds and leaves in a basin of boiling water—about one tablespoon per quart. As soon as the temperature is comfortable, they bathe their feet! Why the feet? Because the heat draws the blood to the lower part of the body, away from the congested areas.

Mustard plaster, a common household remedy for colds and congestion, is used by Gypsies to ease irritation of the kidneys and bladder. They mix one part ground mustard with four parts whole wheat flour, then turn it into a thick paste with warm water. As a precaution against blistering, they may substitute egg whites in place of the water.

There's practically nothing that riles a Gypsy more than the sight of a farmer or gardener destroying plants—*any* plants. "Look at him!" Taras fumed one morning, at one of my uncle's farmhands plowing up the soil. "He destroys life itself!"

"But Taras," I protested, "those are only weeds he's burying."

"*Only* weeds?" He gazed at me incredulously. "It is weeds that have allowed the Gypsy to survive. Weeds in the garden. Weeds in the fields. Even the weeds that creep through cracks in cement!"

His eyes were scanning the ground as we strolled. Suddenly, Taras halted, kneeled, and plucked a lone dandelion. "Behold this weed!" he proclaimed. "Do you know what I am going to do with it, little one? The leaves I shall add to my salad. The roots I shall grind into coffee. And the stem I shall offer to a child with the wart."

I had good cause to remember those words, some weeks later, when small warts sprouted on my hands. "Show me!" my expression read, as I pointed the warts out to Taras.

The old Gypsy led me to a field. Each time we came upon a dandelion, he plucked it and squeezed its stem. When a drop of milky juice exuded, he applied it to a wart. Taras did this over and over, until all my warts were covered with the fast-drying liquid.

"Do not wash it away," he cautioned. "It will vanish by itself. When it does, you must add more. And remember, little one, not to lose patience."

Taras never had a better patient! Not a moment went by, except at night, when my warts weren't caked with dried dandelion milk. One by one, the warts started to turn black, and within three days, they all fell off!

The coffee that Gypsies brew from dandelion roots is not only free of sleep-robbing caffeine, it is actually said to *induce* sleep. It is prepared, first, by roasting the roots until they're brown and hard. The roots are then ground into powder, ready to be brewed like ordinary coffee. Gypsies drink it as both a tonic and a digestive aid.

Neither Taras nor I knew it at the time, but dandelions are rich in vital minerals and vitamins, which they impart to the coffee. The plants, especially the roots, also contain vital alkaloids that soothe and stimulate the digestive organs.

From dandelion leaves, the Gypsies brew a tea which they drink for colds, diabetes, tuberculosis, rheumatism, arthritis, and disorders of the liver, bladder, and kidneys. A strong decoction is drunk to clean the gallbladder and spleen, and to dislodge kidney stones and gallstones. As a blood purifier, contain-

ing many nutritive salts, dandelion—eaten or drunk in any form
—is believed by the Gypsies to normalize high or low blood pressure and to prevent anemia.

I never ceased to marvel at my Gypsy mentor's vast knowledge of medicinal plant-life. He taught me in many ways. Sometimes, he would simply volunteer a piece of information, when he spotted a growth in our path. Like, "Behold the goldenrod, little one! Its leaves, boiled in water, will strengthen the weakest of stomachs."

Often his wisdom had to be solicited. "You wish to cure your cold, you say? Then seek out the ground ivy, which creeps among the hedgerows and along waste ground. Any Gypsy will tell you that its tea cures colds and chases fever."

Occasionally, a simple accident resulted in a long discourse. Like the morning we were out picking berries. . . . "Ouch!" My hand had accidentally closed on a stinging nettle plant. "These darn things are nothing but trouble!"

"Shame on you," Taras chided. "The sting of the nettle is but nothing compared to the pains that it heals."

That day I learned how Gypsies brew a decoction of nettle leaves to cure diarrhea or dysentery, inflamed kidneys, and hemorrhoids. Nettle tea, made from the leaves, rids the lungs and stomach of phlegm and clears excess mucus from the urinary tract.

For any case of internal hemorrhaging, Gypsies drink a strong infusion brewed from the nettle's roots. In cases of difficult external bleeding, they apply boiled leaves to the wound, and this, it is claimed, swiftly stops the flow.

When Taras told me that nettle tea is one of the best remedies for rheumatism, I found it hard to believe—until, many years later, I learned that the plant contains alkaloids that neutralize uric acid. His lauding of the tea for high blood pressure was treated with similar skepticism—until I found out that the nettle is rich in iron, so vital to healthy circulation. The nettle's high vitamin and mineral content also bear out the Gypsies' use of it as a tonic.

Constipation? The Gypsies cure it with nettles-in-milk, boiled. The same concoction is drunk to relieve migraine headaches and halt the vomiting that often accompanies them.

For hives and eczema, Gypsies boil a nettle-leaf decoction until it thickens into a paste, which they rub on the affected area.

Drinking an infusion further helps the condition—and the same infusion, when held in the mouth, heals soreness of the gums, tongue, and throat.

Through the years, as my interest became more serious, I invented a pleasurable game that Taras and I played often. It went something like this . . .

"Taras, how do the Gypsies cure goiter?"

"With bayberry, myrrh, and goldenseal, mixed into water."

"What about gout?"

"A tea brewed from couch grass, which spreads its tentacles everywhere. Also, the burdock, the buckthorn, and the balm of Gilead."

Half the fun was learning the names of strange, exotic plants. The other half came from trying to stump Taras; I never could do this, no matter how rare the disease.

"Taras, give me a cure for scrofula."

"Eat of the plantain, the King's Evil, or the echinacea. Also powerful are the calamus, the coltsfoot, and the vervain."

"Typhoid."

"Bloodroot, yarrow and bitterroot."

"Leprosy."

"Henna leaves, pennyroyal, or queen's delight."

Amazed, I had to keep reminding myself that Gypsies spent many centuries, in many lands, compiling their cures. When one was not available, there was always another to take its place.

"Pleurisy, Taras."

"The butterfly weed, little one, which your people have renamed the 'pleurisy root.' Drinking it, after it has been powdered and steeped in boiling water, will swiftly relieve the pain. It is even more powerful when combined with yarrow, skullcap, or lady's slipper. A pinch of cayenne would not hurt, either."

Sometimes, a personal complaint would bring on the question. "Taras, I'm having a terrible case of hiccoughs. Have you any recommendations?"

"Drink a tea made of the blue cohosh or the black cohosh—or both."

At other times the conditions of an acquaintance produced the question. "My friend's father is always complaining of lumbago, Taras. What do the Gypsies have to say about that?"

"Let him drink copiously the juice of the celery. At the same time he must seek out angelica or rue and drink of their teas."

For many of the conditions that I mentioned, Taras reminded me of an old Gypsy rule of thumb. "In the name of the plant," he said, "can frequently be found the cure. For diseases of the chest, pick the leaves of the chestnut. For the lungs, lungwort. For the liver, liverwort. For the heart, heartsease."

This advice seemed to remind him of something. He thought for a long moment, then asked, "Have you ever seen a Gypsy wearing spectacles, little one?"

I couldn't say that I had.

"And do you know why, little one? Because of eyebright."

He led me to a grassy area, his eyes searching, until he spotted one—an herb about six inches high, with white flowers streaked and spotted with purple and yellow. The next time I felt the slightest eye irritation, Taras advised, steep this eyebright herb in boiling water. After it cooled, I was to strain it and bathe my eyes with it.

The treatment worked the very first time I tried it. Taras gave me that advice more than fifty years ago, and I still have 20-20 vision without glasses. Which is why I cultivate eyebright in my own garden.

Eyebright, Taras also taught me, when taken as a tea, is an ancient Gypsy remedy for faulty memory. (Dried eyebright, for brewing tea, is available in most health-food stores.)

In the years ahead, as a chemistry student and later as a nutritionist, I had many opportunities to study the rare herbs that Gypsies took for granted. Each turned out to have its own medicinal ingredients.

Silverweed, a blood tonic, contains iron, calcium, and magnesium. Calcium is also an ingredient of cleavers, coltsfoot, shepherd's purse, and plantain—all prescribed by the Gypsies for heart troubles. Devils' bit, meadowsweet, and mullein are rich in iron and magnesium.

Many a Gypsy cure is yet to be analyzed in the laboratory. Someday I hope to find out why cowslip tea and mugwort tea really cure insomnia. I have yet to understand why a mixture of scullcap, valerian root, mistletoe, goldenseal root, wahoo bark, hollyhock root, and gentian root all add up to a medicine that strengthens the hair and retards baldness: I only know that I've never met a bald Gypsy!

The list of Gypsy remedies could fill volumes, but Gypsies were very secretive about their medicines and never wrote them down. Only because I was *parnavo*—a friend—did Taras share his wisdom with me. There were some "remedies," however, that he never hid from anyone.

"Fresh air and sunlight are truly medicines," he said. "They feed the body with nourishment as surely as the foods we eat and the liquids we drink. That is why a Gypsy spends his life 'eating' and 'drinking' of the outdoors."

Another Gypsy remedy, he once pointed out, is optimism. "A Gypsy never worries about the day that lies ahead. He is relaxed, his mind and body free of all strain. For a Gypsy knows that as long as he has his health, and the food to keep it, he is richer than any man."

The fields are no longer replete with the marvelous herbs that Taras and I had in our own backyard. Some only grow in remote parts of the world; others have practically vanished—like the Gypsies themselves, who wander the globe in smaller and smaller numbers.

Fewer, too, are the seekers of nature's cures. On land where herbs once grew, free to anyone, chemical factories produce costly synthetic compounds, while tainting the Gypsies' favorite medicines—sunlight and air—with poisonous fumes.

"Tell me, little one, what is it that all men are doing at the same time?"

"I don't know. Tell me, Taras."

"They grow older."

And then, as an afterthought, he said, "If only they grew wiser, too."

GYPSY REMEDIES FROM AROUND THE WORLD

Convulsions or Fits

> peony
> black-cherry water
> spirit of hart-horn

Mix equal quantities of peony and black-cherry water. Add spirit of hart-horn: five drops for a child, thirty drops for a man, twenty drops for a woman.

Drink during or before a fit.

Complexion

rosemary flowers
white wine

Boil flowers in wine and use as a face wash.
Drink it to sweeten the breath.

Cough Syrup

1 ounce horseradish root
3 ounces horehound
3 cups water
½ cup honey

Simmer horseradish and horehound in boiling water until liquid is reduced to half. Strain and add honey.
Dose: One to two teaspoonfuls as needed.

Dizziness

2 drams broom-wart
2 drams dried chamomile
ivy juice
oil of roses
white wine

Mix above with equal parts ivy juice, oil of roses, and white wine until it turns into a thick salve. Place on a soft cloth and bind to the temples.

Earache

oil of roses
vinegar
chamomile
melilot

Mix small quantity of oil of roses and vinegar and put it into the ear. Make a small bag of soft gauze with equal amounts of chamomile and melilot and place it over the ear.

Freckles and Blotches

> wild cucumber roots
> narcissus roots
> strong brandy

Dry equal amounts of wild cucumber roots and narcissus roots in the shade, then reduce to a very fine powder. Add this to strong brandy and wash the face with it until it begins to itch. Then wash with cold water. Repeat daily.

Kidney Stones

> hot milk
> wine
> chamomile flowers

Make a drink of hot milk and wine, take off the curd and add a handful of chamomile flowers. Place into a pewter pot and let stand on a hot stove until it dissolves.

Dose: Drink as often as necessary.

Liniment

> 1 tablespoon horseradish root
> ½ cup oil

Grate horseradish root in a cup and pour boiling oil over it. Let cool to a bearable temperature and rub the painful areas with it or apply as a compress. Bottle what is left for future use.

Lip Salve

> 1 ounce myrrh
> 1 ounce litharge powder
> 4 ounces honey
> 2 ounces beeswax
> 6 ounces oil of roses

Mix ingredients well over a slow fire. Let cool and apply as necessary.

Nosebleed

> 1 egg white
> rose water
> powdered alabaster

Beat egg white; add rose water and powdered alabaster. Dip flax in the concoction and place on the temples two or three times a day.

Sore Mouth
or Gums

> 40 drops spirit of vitriol
> 1 ounce honey of roses

Mix ingredients well. Keep moistening sore as long as necessary.

Sore Throat

> 1 egg white
> ½ plantain
> ½ pint rose water
> 4 teaspoons houseleek juice
> 20 drops vitriol
> 1 ounce honey of roses

Beat egg white into plantain and rose water. Add the rest of the ingredients. Gargle as often as necessary.

Sores
(External)

> elder leaves
> milk

Boil elder leaves (handful) in milk until they are soft. Strain them and boil again until mixture thickens. Place on sore as often as necessary.

Tonic

> ¼ ounce horseradish root
> 2 ounces celery root (or chopped fresh celery)
> 1 ounce dandelion root
> 2 pints water

Place roots in a saucepan and bring to a boil. Reduce heat, cover, and let simmer twenty minutes. Strain and bottle.
Dose: A wineglassful twice a day.

Wrinkles

> 2 ounces juice of white lily roots
> 2 ounces fine honey
> 1 ounce melted white wax

Mix ingredients well.
Apply every night and do not remove until morning.

Quiet Rest

> red roses
> violets
> melilot
> ½ dram white poppy
> ½ dram white henbane
> dillsfeet

Take a handful of red roses, violets, and melilot; combine with other ingredients and put all in a soft linen cloth about twelve inches long and three inches wide. Then tie this to the forehead.

10

Garlic: The Natural Antibiotic

Are you old enough to remember the great flu epidemic of 1918? It was a year of terror across the land. Victims died by the score, and of those who survived, many were left with permanent respiratory weakness or with brains damaged by high fever. Back then, medical science had little to offer in the way of protection.

When the first outbreaks occurred, my grandmother summoned the family into solemn council. Grandma, always good for a quip or two, barely cracked a smile as she greeted each arrival. This was one of her rare moments—stern and serious.

"Children," she announced when we were all assembled, "I'll get right down to business." Briefly, Grandma recounted news reports of the spreading flu, and then she produced a large bundle. "In here," she said, "is the medicine that'll protect us."

She upended the bundle and out poured the "medicine": garlic—what looked like a ton of it. "You're each to take a handful," Grandma ordered. "And until the epidemic passes, Lord help the one I catch without a piece of garlic in his mouth!"

My grandmother meant it. The year 1918 was a garlicky year in our family. Garlic was added to our soups, salads, and meats— and sometimes even to our beverages. Between meals we chewed on bits of garlic, and at night we slept with pieces tucked between our gums and cheeks. Grandma never eased up. Not a day passed without some sort of reminder—a surprise visit, a phone call, even a postcard.

But who could fault her fierce tenacity? Influenza struck our community as it did the rest of the country. Schools were closed down. CONTAGION signs appeared on houses all over town. Many close friends were bedridden for weeks, and some never recovered.

As for our own family, not a single case occurred. Indeed, the flu epidemic passed us by without causing so much as a sniffle.

Actually, my grandmother wasn't merely trying out some personal whim when she put us on a garlic regimen. During that same period, garlic came into great demand everywhere. The price skyrocketed; many people, including doctors, were paying a dollar a pound for it.

Was this some national fad, born of desperation? How do today's "wonder" drugs stack up against garlic as a flu preventive?

In 1965, when a flu outbreak threatened Russia, the government flew in a 500-ton emergency supply of garlic. The Soviets, whose scientists had already done extensive research on garlic, ran notices in the Moscow *Evening Journal,* advising citizens to eat more garlic because of "its prophylactic qualities for preventing flu."

During the London flu epidemic that traveled halfway around the world in the winter of 1972–1973, thousands of deaths were reported in major European cities. At the height of the epidemic came this Associated Press news item, dated February 15, 1973:

ITALY FLU EPIDEMIC REPORTED TO BE MILD

ROME (AP)—The flu epidemic has reached Italy, but in a mild form that has not spread nationwide, the Health Ministry said Tuesday . . . In Southern Italy, a few isolated cases have been reported.

Italy, as everyone knows, is a nation of garlic eaters.

The medicinal use of garlic has a centuries-old history that goes back to 3000 B.C. Babylonians used it as both food and medicine, and so did the ancient Greeks, Romans, Hebrews, Arabians, Egyptians, and many other Far Eastern and Middle Eastern peoples.

Muhammad recommended garlic to his followers for both internal and external use. Hippocrates prescribed it for intestinal complaints and infectious diseases. Galen, the Roman physician whose teachings dominated medicine for more than a thousand

years, called garlic an "antidote to poison," while his country-
man, Pliny, believed it could cure respiratory, bronchial, and
tubercular conditions. When Dioscorides was official physician
of the Roman army, he prescribed garlic as a vermifuge (worm
expellant) and as a remedy for all respiratory and intestinal ailments.

When the Great Plague swept through Europe in the four-
teenth century, it was recorded that those who ate regular, substantial amounts of garlic escaped the dreaded "black death."
During the seventeenth-century Great Plague of London, Daniel
Defoe, in his *Journal of the Plague Year,* and Samuel Pepys, in
his famed *Diary,* immortalized one family that completely escaped infection. Their home, dubbed "God's Provident House,"
contained vast stores of garlic in the kitchen and cellar. When
another plague struck Marseilles, France, in the eighteenth
century, a garlic-vinegar preparation, called the "Four Thieves,"
was consumed for protection.

In more recent times, the British government, during World
War I, bought thousands of tons of garlic to treat wounded soldiers returning from the front. And as late as World War II, the
Russians placed peeled, cut cloves of garlic around the edges
of battle-wounds to speed healing and check infection.

Before diphtheria came under the control of vaccination, an
ancient Middle Eastern remedy consisted of keeping a small,
peeled garlic clove in the mouth day and night, except when
sleeping or eating. Every so often the patient was to give a light
nibble or crunch to release the juice. After the clove was chewed
down to a nub or pulp, it was immediately replaced with a
fresh one.

When Arab children are struck by whooping cough, their
mothers feed them ten to twenty drops of garlic juice in syrup or
honey, every four hours. For the rare adult who contracts this
disease, a small bottle or jar is half-filled with freshly chopped,
slightly macerated garlic, and used as an inhaler—frequent and
prolonged. When not in use, the container is kept tightly covered, so the volatile, penetrating vapors will retain their
strength.

In lesser dosages, these garlic treatments are still widely used
as remedies for colds, for nasal, sinus, or chest congestion, and
for throat infections. The rule to remember, if you try them in

your own home, is to renew the garlic preparation before it completely loses its potency.

Is there any basis for garlic's curative claims, or are they merely unsubstantiated forms of "faith healing"? Modern science may already have answered this question.

The active factor in garlic is a chemical called *allicin*. Unlike commercial antibiotics, which destroy friendly bacteria along with the virulent ones, allicin wipes out only the dangerous germs. But instead of killing the germs instantly, garlic uses a suffocating effect on them. The allicin and other chemicals in garlic oil unite with virus matter and inactivate it by destroying the germs' oxygen metabolism. In effect, close contact with garlic literally asphyxiates the germs.

Sometimes called Russian penicillin, the antibiotic power of garlic has been harnessed by Russian clinics in the form of volatile oils or extracts called *phitoncides*. For most disorders, the patient simply inhales these phitoncides. Extracted from garlic and other plants known to possess anti-infection properties, phitoncides are powerful, natural germ killers. Their concentrated effect is so potent that even a small amount has a devastating effect on disease bacteria.

When Russian peasants develop minor ear troubles—aches, buzzing, infections—they peel a clove of garlic and insert it in the ear, holding it in place with a plug of cotton. In Leningrad clinics, infections of the middle ear are treated with direct applications of garlic phitoncides to the diseased tissues. Nasal infections are also treated with local applications of this concentrated garlic extract.

Taking their lead from folk usages throughout the land, Soviet doctors claim remarkable results from the inhalation of garlic extracts. Not only do these doctors use them for the usual range of nasal and respiratory infections, but also for the treatment of intestinal disorders and high blood pressure. Even tubercular patients seem to recover more rapidly when garlic inhalations are added to their regular treatment.

To one who has surveyed folk medicine around the world, none of these treatments comes as startling news. Truly astonishing, however, was a garlic-cure I witnessed during a fact-finding tour of Iranian Azerbaijan.

Walking past a native hut, I sensed the familiar aroma of

simmering garlic. Though Iranians are not noted for their use of garlic in cookery, the smell was overpowering, almost dizzying. My curiosity was whetted: What possible dish could contain all that garlic?

It wasn't food they were cooking; it was medicine. Entering the hut, I saw a young girl lying on straw matting. Her choking and wheezing and her feverish, swollen eyes showed all the outward symptoms of pneumonia. In an old iron saucepan on an ancient stone stove, the sizzling mass of garlic sent out colorless fumes that made the room dance before my rapidly tearing eyes.

Heady from the scent, I watched the girl's mother at the stove. Every so often she poured some hot garlic juice onto a long, wide strip of cotton. When the cotton was thoroughly soaked and slightly cooled, she turned it over to the girl's father, who laid it on his daughter's heaving chest. Each time the compress lost its warmth, it was replaced by a fresh one.

The father also placed small wads of soaked cotton in the girl's nose and ears, replacing these, too, when they turned cool. At the same time, he gently fed her small bits of grated garlic.

Suddenly, the child began to cough. In that same instant, the father turned her quickly on her side. The coughing was soon followed by instinctive hawking from deep down in the lungs. Next came a torrent of mucus from her mouth and nose, while her eyes gushed profusely.

Nobody except myself seemed worried, and I soon realized why. The coughing and expectorating lasted for only a minute or so, but in that brief time the girl's breathing became smooth and even, her eyelids closed comfortably. A faint smile of relief graced her lips, as she turned on her back and swiftly fell into a deep sleep.

It isn't often that one has the opportunity to observe such dramatic cures firsthand. Afterward, as I continued my tour through this ancient land, I frequently came upon natives with mouths puckered up like chipmunks. One whiff was enough to tell me that their cheeks were loaded with garlic. This was their age-old remedy for respiratory ailments, infected tonsils and sinuses, laryngitis, pharyngitis, and bronchitis.

Are these also fanciful folk fantasies? Here are some findings of Dr. Kristine Nolti, a physician at the Humlegaarden health resort in Humlebaek, Denmark: "At Humlegaarden, epidemic colds are unknown. Everyone knows he must use garlic when a cold begins. If one puts a piece of garlic in his mouth, at the onset of a cold, on both sides between the cheeks and teeth, the cold will disappear within a few hours or, at most, within a day."

Dr. Nolti recommends this same treatment for the conditions I encountered among my Iranian friends, and also for catarrh and for chronic inflammation of the salivary glands and neighboring lymph glands. As in the ancient treatment for diphtheria, the garlic must be kept in the mouth constantly, except when eating or sleeping, and renewed when it loses its potency.

Descendants of the Yugoslav Macedonians have added their own variation to garlic therapy for colds and related infections: an eighth of an ounce of garlic juice in a cup of beef tea, bouillon, or other liquid, three to four times a day. This same drink, also taken to reduce fevers, was later adapted by Dr. Albert Schweitzer at his jungle clinic in French Equatorial Africa.

As a remedy for asthma, farmers in the south of England add several cloves of raw garlic to their food each day. Or they drink comfrey tea with two cloves added to each cupful. This last decoction may taste more like garlic than like comfrey, but each ingredient has the reputation of relieving asthmatic symptoms.

Paris in the spring may conjure up romantic visions to some, but since the sixteenth century, the coming of spring is a signal for Parisians and provincial Frenchmen to eat lots of garlic and butter for two or three weeks. This annual custom may be on the wane, but some of my French friends still observe it religiously. They believe that it improves their health for the rest of the year.

If you're counting calories or limiting your cholesterol consumption, you can derive the same benefits of this spring tonic by mixing the garlic into a vinegar and salad oil dressing. Or you can substitute an American farm version, which consists of chopped garlic, dark molasses, and powdered flowers of sulfur.

Need a memory jogger? When Mrs. Eleanor Roosevelt, at a late age, was asked the secret of her remarkable memory, she replied, "Garlic cloves." Having read that garlic was an ancient folk remedy for failing memory, Mrs. Roosevelt faithfully consumed three honey-covered cloves every morning. Modern naturopaths claim that the same benefits can be derived by eating garlic raw in salads and taking boosters of garlic perles, the tiny capsules that have no taste and leave no odor on the breath.

High blood pressure, an ailment that crops up nearly everywhere, has been treated with garlic by many folk peoples. In the Indian state of Goa, natives carry small bottles of garlic juice, from which they take a nip whenever they feel the pressure starting to rise. Tribesmen of Medes, at the first sign of rising blood pressure, chew vigorously on bits of garlic until pressure returns to normal. The Menangkabaus of Indonesia do the same with grated garlic.

Dr. F. G. Piotrowski, a member of the medical faculty at the University of Geneva, has added some scientific weight to this unique use of garlic. Experimenting with one hundred hypertensive patients, whom he treated with garlic oil, Dr. Piotrowski reported that an average drop of two centimeters in blood pressure occurred within a week of garlic therapy. Symptoms of dizziness, headache, and angina-like pains were relieved within three to five days after treatment began. He recommended that doctors include garlic capsules in their standard treatment of hypertension.

Wherever garlic is eaten as medicine, it is also used externally as a treatment for numerous skin conditions, ranging from infected pimples to precancerous lesions, ulcerations, and thickened patches of the skin. This has led to tests at Humlegaarden, where even the worst pimples, according to Dr. Nolti, "disappear without leaving a scar, if rubbed several times daily with garlic."

More significant was an experiment conducted at the District Ontological Dispensary in Kirovograd, Russia. Dr. D. M. Sergeiev and Dr. I. D. Leonov made a paste by rubbing garlic in a mortar until it was reduced to pulp. It was then placed on gauze and applied, from eight to twelve hours, on one hundred and ninety-four precancerous conditions of the lip and mouth. The two scientists reported complete healing in over 90 percent of the cases.

A warning was added, however: Home treatment should not be attempted until diagnosis has shown that the condition is merely *pre*cancerous, not an actual cancer that requires professional treatment.

The peasants of Sardinia have handed down a simple garlic remedy for one of mankind's most nettlesome problems—mosquito bites. Before venturing out into mosquito territory, they eat a big salad dripping with garlic dressing. Or, if they're not hungry, they rub the dressing over all exposed parts of their bodies.

Mosquitos, it's been proven, hate garlic—maybe because they recognize an "enemy" when they smell it. Biologist Eldon L. Reeves, of the University of California, tested garlic extract on five species of mosquitos. Mortality was 100 percent!

What comes as a great surprise to most people is garlic's use, throughout antiquity, as a remedy for indigestion. If anything, garlic is often blamed for *causing* digestive disorders because its strong flavor masks the taste of the foods that are really the cause. Many folk people know better.

Lepcha mothers, in Bhutan, soothe their colicky infants by placing minute grains of garlic on their tongues. When a Kuban Cossack senses an approaching bout with nausea or dyspepsia, he quickly belts down a clove or two. The Tibetans attack these same complaints with garlic juice added to milk of the yak.

Garlic's effectiveness against digestive troubles was recently confirmed by Dr. Harry Barowsky and Dr. Linn J. Boyd. In the *Review of Gastroenterology,* they described their use of garlic capsules in testing fifty patients who suffered from "various disorders commonly associated with gastrointestinal symptoms."

The conditions described were indigestion, discomfort after meals, gas, abdominal distention, nausea, and vomiting. While they were taking garlic, their improvement was so marked, and followed such a regular pattern, that the doctors stated, "This remedy should merit consideration in treatment when these symptoms [of gastric distress] are present." Their findings were later confirmed by Dr. F. Damran and Dr. E. A. Ferguson, who concluded that garlic has a sedative effect on the stomach.

Perhaps the best summation of garlic's medicinal qualities was made by Dr. Nolti, who declared, "Garlic has a strengthening and laxative effect, lowers too high blood pressure and raises one which is too low. It also cures indigestion, disinfects the contents of the stomachs of those who lack hydrochloric acid in their gastric juices for this purpose, kills putrefaction bacteria in the large intestine, and neutralizes poisons in the organism itself."

With all these virtues going for it, is there any wonder that in

Central Rumania (the legendary land known as Transylvania), some natives still believe that garlic even has the power to repel werewolves? The lesson is clear: The next time you catch a whiff of garlic, don't turn your nose up at it—unless you happen to be a werewolf!

GARLIC REMEDIES FROM AROUND THE WORLD

Aching Joints
Deep-Heat Garlic Ointment—From England

> ¾ cup garlic, minced or finely chopped
> 1 cup pure lard

Put both ingredients in a jar and set the jar in a pan of boiling water. Stir occasionally as the lard melts. Let stand in the boiling water for three hours, renewing the water when necessary to keep the pan from boiling dry. Remove from fire and let cool until the mixture solidifies. Stir well. Cover tightly until ready to use.

Massage on stiff and aching joints. This ointment can also be used as a penetrating rub for chest colds, bronchitis, lung congestion, and related ailments.

Colds and Coughs
Garlic Cold and Cough Remedy—From Poland

> ½ cup honey
> 1 tablespoon chopped garlic
> 1 teaspoon horseradish (fresh, scraped root is preferred; if not available, use prepared)

Mix well and take one or two teaspoonfuls as needed. If mixture is too hot, add more honey to taste.

Eczema and Skin Irritations
Garlic Skin Salve—From Russia

> zinc-oxide ointment
> lanolin
> garlic powder

Mix equal parts of zinc-oxide ointment and lanolin until thoroughly blended. Add equal amount of garlic powder a little at a time to prevent lumping and caking. When the mixture is blended smoothly, store in a covered jar and use as required. (Zinc-oxide ointment and lanolin are available in drugstores, and garlic powder in health-food stores and supermarkets.)

Hemorrhoids
Garlic Skin Salve—From Russia

For uncomplicated hemorrhoids, use the above Garlic Skin Salve as a healing external application. For internal application, remove dry outer skin from garlic clove, scrape clove to allow juice to exude. Insert into rectum as a suppository when retiring and allow to remain in the body all night. It will be expelled the next day through the process of normal elimination. Repeat as needed.

Intestinal Parasites
Worm Remedy—From Pakistan

2 or 3 cloves garlic
1 glass warm water

Peel and chop garlic cloves very fine. Drop into a standard-size water glass and add warm water. The glass should be about two-thirds full. Stir, cover, and let stand overnight. Stir mixture again in the morning and let garlic settle to the bottom, or strain, then drink the water.

Insect Repellent
Insect Repellent Oil—From France

1 cup safflower oil or sesame-seed oil
½ cup feverfew (bachelor's button)
blossoms or 1 tablespoon, dried
8 cloves chopped garlic

Simmer safflower or sesame-seed oil with feverfew blossoms or dried feverfew for twenty minutes. Remove from fire, cool slightly, and add garlic cloves well chopped. Pour into a wide-mouthed bottle or jar and let stand a week, shaking mixture two or three times a day. Strain. Apply to the skin as an insect repellent, or as a remedy for bites when you forget to use it in advance.

11

Some Rediscovered Germ Killers

As any historian will tell you, the world of folk medicine abounds with hearsay and rumors. One can spend a lifetime tracking down reports of wise old healers and their miracle cures. More often than not, their claims prove to be grossly exaggerated if not downright deceptive. Separating folk-fact from folk-fiction requires a great deal of healthy curiosity, tempered by a liberal dose of skepticism.

It was this attitude that brought me to a tiny village in the French Alps, many years ago. My host was a physician of that community, a man with a wondrous reputation. Rumor had it that he could cure any number of infections—influenza, mastoiditis, blood poisoning—you name it! And this was in an era before the discovery of antibiotics. Could you blame me for being more than a little skeptical?

His medical armamentarium proved even more curious. The doctor, a hale and hearty octogenarian, kept a storeroom full of breads and cheeses, which, he explained, were the source of his marvelous medicine.

And what was this "medicine"? *Mold!* The very same mold that forms on your bread and other foods if you leave them exposed too long. The mold that the world's great cheesemakers use to create their delicacies.

Each morning the doctor carefully scraped accumulated mold into a glass receptacle, sealed it, and let it stand for a few days. Still demanding positive proof, I accompanied him on house-calls, where he administered the green, foul-smelling mold, sparingly, to patients wracked with congestion, coughing, and high fever.

Before long I had to admit that I'd never witnessed such speedy recoveries. Fevers responded almost instantly to the mold-treatment. Infections known to be fatal—or to hang on for weeks, at best—were reduced in a matter of days. Convinced that I'd witnessed an authentic cure, I asked the doctor why he didn't publicize his discovery and encourage its use in every household? His answer proved prophetic.

The mold, he explained, contained some substance with the power to kill harmful bacteria. But there was danger in using it too much and too often—the danger of creating new, stronger strains of bacteria, able to resist the power of mold. Until science could isolate and understand the unknown substance in mold, he preferred to keep his cure a private matter.

Science, as most of us now know, did indeed uncover the answer to mold's healing powers, for it is from mold that laboratories extract the most famous of modern antibiotics, penicillin. And for the reasons predicted by the French doctor, penicillin—and other antibiotics—are in danger of being used indiscriminately . . . not by the average person but by the medical profession itself.

Germ-fighting folk remedies go back for centuries, long before man even suspected the existence of bacteria. Some of these cures, like the garlic, have had a rebirth in scientific circles. Others have been overlooked or neglected to a point where they're all but forgotten.

Medicine men of the Cree tribes, for example, relied on an herb called pipsissewa to cure a variety of ailments. So powerful was its action against tuberculosis, scrofula, and rheumatism that it later became one of the regular medicines used by frontier doctors. Among the Indians, pipsissewa tea was drunk at the first signs of urinary infection—diseases that the White Man's medicine later labeled as nephritis, urethritis, and cystitis. According to research described in the *Canadian Journal of Botany*, extracts from two hundred and nine separate plants were recently tested for their antibacterial properties. Pipsissewa proved to be one of the most potent.

In the sixteenth century the herb sassafras was perhaps the

most widely used medicine throughout Europe. It had been brought to the continent by explorers who first discovered its amazing curative properties among the American Indians. The Seminoles drank sassafras tea to relieve coughs, the pain of gallstones, and bladder irritations. The Rappahannocks brewed an infusion of sassafras roots, to bring out the rash of measles and as a fever reducer. From the shoots of sassafras plants, Mohawk medicine men extracted the pith and soaked it in water. After straining it, they used it as a bath for inflamed eyes. Iroquois tribesmen brewed a decoction from the root-bark, with which they treated rheumatism and ailments of the bladder, kidney, and throat. The Iroquois also considered this drink a tonic after childbirth, a blood purifier, and a tonic for the stomach and bowels.

Early in this century, scientists became intrigued by the fact that people who drank sassafras tea appeared to have a higher-than-average resistance to colds and throat infections. In laboratories the bark of the root yielded a number of substances possessing antiseptic powers. A scientific breakthrough was in the making, when World War I broke out, causing a suspension of research. By the time study could be resumed, the medical world had shifted its sight to the burgeoning new field of antibiotic drugs.

"Purge me with hyssop, and I shall be clean. Wash me, and I shall be whiter than snow." Thus spoke King David (Psalms 51:7) of an ancient herb whose use as a medicine has all but vanished. So potent were the curative properties of hyssop that it became a symbol of purification from sin.

In ancient Babylonia, hyssop tea was drunk to reduce fever and applied to the eyes to cure infections. The Babylonians also used hyssop for colds and chest infections, and as a gargle for sore throats. Levantine tribesmen found that hyssop could lower blood pressure, relieve the kidneys and bladder (by inducing perspiration), and remedy such diverse conditions as jaundice and epilepsy. Wherever hyssop was used medicinally, it was also applied externally to kill lice and brewed into a decoction to expel worms.

In some small pockets of the Middle East, hyssop is still a household remedy. Little are those "primitives" aware of a recent scientific discovery—that hyssop leaves grow the mold that produces penicillin!

At the same time that Asians were relying on hyssop, tribesmen of Africa found many of the same properties in another near-forgotten herb, elecampane. Before being naturalized in the New World, this versatile plant was used by the Diolas to warm and strengthen the lungs and to relieve bronchial infections. Combined with other herbs, it was also effective against tuberculosis.

Afterward, when elecampane's reputation had spread, the root was sucked or chewed by asthmatic Londoners whenever they traveled in polluted areas. It soon became an ingredient of syrups and lozenges for coughs and colds, asthma, bronchitis, and catarrh.

Elecampane, it was later learned, contains an alkaloid called heleninum. One part of this powerful antibiotic and antiseptic, in ten thousand parts of water, can instantly kill ordinary bacteria.

As science continues to rediscover the medicinal value of various foods, the list of antibiotic plants grows by leaps and bounds. In the avocado seed has been found a potent germ-killing substance. Wheat and barley juice contain a number of antibiotics. Substances resembling penicillin have been isolated from seeds of the ash, dog rose, honey locust, privet, and white acacia.

High on the list of rediscovered medicinal folk-foods is the common garden sage. Used primarily today in sauces and dressings, this worldwide plant, in all its varieties, has a long history of medicinal application. Hippocrates described its use to combat a pestilence in Egypt. John Wesley prescribed it as a cure for palsy, while Father Sebastian Kneipp recommended it for ailing liver and kidneys and for wounds that resist healing.

Deep in the African interior, the natives have a unique cure for infected tonsils. A hot sage poultice is wrapped around the throat, and on top of it is placed another wrapping to retain the heat. As soon as the poultice starts cooling, it's replaced by a fresh one. At the same time the patient gargles frequently with an infusion brewed from the sage plant. This treatment continues without break until the swelling and inflammation subside—usually in a few hours, rarely longer than a full day.

Still prevalent among German farm women is the use of sage tea to wean their infants from breast-feeding. When the breasts grow sore and inflamed, indicating that the time has come for weaning, the mother drinks large quantities of sage tea. This not only heals the breast troubles but also halts production of milk.

Indians of the Rocky Mountains drank hot sage tea to stimulate perspiration and cold sage tea to stimulate the kidneys and bladder. Greek Cypriots still treat laryngitis, pharyngitis, tonsillitis, and ulcerated tongue or mouth with a small glassful of sage infusion, swallowed three times a day. For these same conditions, and also for fevers, British farmers pour hot vinegar over sage leaves, add water, and drink or gargle with it.

Modern herbalists, especially in Europe, use sage extracts as mouthwashes to heal bleeding gums and to halt excessive flow of saliva. Concentrated sage is also prescribed as a remedy for mental exhaustion or for hypersensitivity. Oral thrush, a fungus disease of the mouth, regresses rapidly when bathed in sage tea.

Recent experiments have shown that sage contains a large number of antiseptic substances, and its oils are able to destroy bacteria. Sage's antibiotic properties are even showing themselves effective against bacteria that resist penicillin. All the evidence, to date, indicates that hidden in sage are a number of germ killers yet to be exposed.

The same is true of one of the commonest foods in our vegetable bins: the onion. Prized as a folk remedy for thousands of years, its healing powers are barely remembered in the kitchens of present-day "wonder-drug" cultures. But in some parts of England and other European countries, the natives still swear by a most novel use of onion. Whenever an epidemic threatens—be it flu, measles, chicken pox, or scarlet fever—they peel onions, cut them in half, and hang them in every room of the house. The onions are said to absorb any germs floating in the air.

After twelve hours they hang fresh onions and burn the old ones. Never eat an onion that has been exposed, they warn, for you may wind up eating the very germs that you were trying to trap.

Another English cold and flu preventive is hot onion broth combined with an equal amount of catnip tea. The tea is steeped in a covered teapot for five minutes, then added to the hot broth. *Dose:* a cupful three or four times a day and especially before retiring. A French variation is hot onion soup liberally laced with slivers of garlic, taken in the same dosages. Frenchmen also chew on raw onion to keep the mouth and throat germ-free.

For inflamed mucous membrane, sinusitis, and head colds, the Ghegs of Albania simmer fenugreek seeds in water for thirty minutes. After straining the tea, they add a tablespoon of onion juice and two teaspoons of lemon juice to each cupful. They drink at least two cupfuls a day—before bedtime and upon awakening—and more as needed.

Spanish farmers treat pleurisy with a poultice of sliced or chopped onion, heated to a comfortable temperature but not cooked. The same poultice is used for chest colds, while a smaller version, applied to abscesses and boils, is reputed to draw out the infection, reduce inflammation, and speed healing.

Natives of Africa's Ivory Coast apply onion juice to burns and scalds, to prevent infection and blistering. In Greece a slice of lemon is dipped in olive oil, then rubbed gently over minor burns, or applied as a poultice to severe ones.

Throughout Africa, hot roasted onions are used to relieve earaches and minor infections of the ear. Wrapped in cloth, the onion is placed over the ear until it cools, then is replaced with a freshly roasted one. Treatment continues until the condition abates.

Back to England for an old remedy for congestion of the chest or lungs: chopped onion combined with the gray lichen (called "lungs of oak") growing on oak trees. Two tablespoons of the lichen are boiled in two cups of water for twenty minutes. Just before it is removed from the fire, a half cup of chopped onion is added. The resulting decoction is covered, allowed to stand until cool, then strained. When ready to use, it's reheated to a comfortable warmth, then applied as a compress or massaged vigorously on the chest and over the lungs.

When my cousin John and I were about seven years old, we went to spend some of our summer vacation with Grandma. No sooner did we arrive than John came down with a summer cold and fever. That night Grandma fed us some raw onion, then sent us to bed. The next morning, when I went into John's room, his cold and fever were gone, and Grandma was removing woolen socks from his feet.

"I smell cooked onions," I announced.

"Of course you do," Grandma replied, shaking some peeled slivers from the socks. "See? Instead of cooking Johnny, the fever cooked the onions!"

Years later I learned that binding slices of onion to the soles is an old Italian remedy for feverish colds. Held in place by woolen socks, the onion is believed to draw off both infection and fever by morning.

As a relative latecomer to the field of modern research, the onion has demonstrated some amazing properties to bolster her ancient claims. Britain's Dr. Eric Powell, who verified nearly all of these claims, also recommends onions—raw, cooked, or potentized—for urinary weakness. "They act as a tonic," he stated, "to the bladder sphincter muscle."

A German physician, Dr. J. Klosa, was among the early experimenters with both garlic and onion. Writing in the *German Medical Monthly,* he told of using a combination of garlic oil and fresh extract of onion juice on patients suffering from grippe, sore throat, and rhinitis. Previously Dr. Klosa had experimented with garlic oil alone, but he found that when onion juice was added, there were no post-grippe complications. Patients recovered much more rapidly, without developing such secondary symptoms as throat and ear infections, chronic inflammation of the lungs and bronchi, swelling of the lymph glands, and intestinal disorders.

Switzerland's Dr. Alfred Vogel suggests two onion remedies for head colds. One is simply to cut an onion in half and place the halves on a bedside table near your head, so you can inhale the fumes while you sleep. The other is to place a thick slice of raw onion in a glass, pour boiling water over it, let stand a few seconds, remove the onion and drink the water.

In India a mixture of onion juice and honey is prescribed for coughs and colds—and also as a remedy for seminal weakness in males. Indian folk physicians prescribe onion-juice nose drops not only for colds and sinus troubles but also as a treatment for nosebleed. And instead of smelling salts, Indian women take a few strong whiffs of onion to counteract dizziness and fainting spells.

Wherein lies the antibiotic powers of onion? Russian electro-
biologists may have found the answer in an ultraviolet emission
of onions called *mitogenic radiation* (M Rays). These radiations appear to stimulate cell activity and rejuvenate the entire
system. M Rays are also emitted by garlic and ginseng. *Most
important of all, however, is the finding that an electrical field,
similar to M Rays, is emitted by penicillin.*

Yet another breakthrough is in the making. After ten years of
research and experimentation, Dr. Nikolai Kharchenko, director of pharmacology at Kharkov Medical Institute, reports
the successful use of onion in heart and circulatory disorders.
The basis for this claim is allicepum, a substance that the
Russians have extracted from onions. Allicepum has been found
especially helpful for patients with weak hearts, high blood
pressure, and hardening of the arteries. It reduces cholesterol
and markedly improves circulation in the arteries, the vital
vessels that carry the blood to the heart. This effect, in turn,
strengthens the action of the heart.

Though allicepum is not available outside of Russia, onions
certainly are. Dr. Kharchenko believes strongly in a moderate
but regular daily intake of onions, in some form, for optimum
health. "Onion is beneficial to people of all ages," he says,
"including those who have lived to advanced age. It is *essential*
to include onions in the daily diet."

I couldn't help recalling this statement when I was doing
research on longevity in Bulgaria. Interviewing Dobry Kaloyan,
a one-hundred-and-six-year-old who still held a full-time job, I
asked what was responsible for the long, healthy lives of himself
and his countrymen.

Dobry responded with the usual reasons given for the Bul-
garians' longevity. "We stay active, work hard all our lives, eat
plain, wholesome food, but not to stuff ourselves. And we sleep
with mostly clear conscience—except sometimes."

"What about you, personally?" I went on. "Is there any *one
thing* that you think has contributed to your long life?"

"One thing?" Dobry scratched his head in thought, then
nodded. "One thing I do steady is eat an onion every day, as I
have all my life. *An onion every single day!*"

With all the evidence in favor of it, I intend to do the same.
What about you?

GERM-KILLING FOLK RECIPES

**Colds,
Coughs,
Sore Throat**

Sage Gargle—From Greece

1 ounce sage
1 dram (⅛ ounce) cayenne powder
1 pint water

Bring water to a boil. Add ingredients and steep for twelve hours. Use as needed.

Onion-Honey-Pine Cough Syrup—From Sweden

1 cup honey
1 cup water
½ cup chopped onion
⅓ cup pine-tree buds

Mix honey and water. Add other ingredients and bring to a boil. Reduce heat, cover, and simmer slowly for twenty minutes.

Dose: Adults, one tablespoon; children, one to two teaspoons, as needed.

Onion-Honey-Flaxseed Cough Syrup—From Mexico

1 tablespoon flaxseed
3 cups water
⅔ cup finely chopped onion
½ cup honey
¼ cup lemon juice

Simmer flaxseed in water until liquid is reduced to half. Remove from fire and stir in onion and honey. Cool and add lemon juice.

Dose: Adults, one tablespoon; children 1 to 2 teaspoons. Don't swallow immediately. Chew first, since onions kill germs in mouth and throat.

Skin Diseases

Sassafras Brew—From American Indians

$\frac{1}{2}$ ounce sassafras bark
2 ounces red clover flowers
1 ounce burdock root
1 ounce blue flag root
1 pint water

Place all ingredients in water and bring to a boil. Simmer for twenty minutes and strain when cool.

Dose: One wineglassful three times daily, as long as necessary.

12

Medical Magic from the Beehive

Wide-eyed with wonderment, the boy brought his veiled face close to the beehive and listened for a long moment. "I never heard such loud buzzing," he said. "They sure sound mad this morning. Is something bothering them, Mr. Mulholland?"

Through the fine wire-mesh guarding his own face, the tall white-haired man smiled, and in a voice feigning disapproval, he said, "Lelord, what did you have for breakfast?"

"Onion omelette."

"That explains it."

"Explains what, Mr. Mulholland?"

"Why the bees are angry, Lelord. Strange odors upset them, and they're quick to let you know it. They're telling you to quit breathing that onion all over their hive."

To an eight-year-old boy, just starting to learn the mysteries of nature, that was a fascinating discovery. Just as fascinating was the tiny stove, mounted on a pair of bellows, which Mr. Mulholland brought to the mouth of the hive. "Won't that make them even madder?" the boy asked.

"Nope," replied Mr. Mulholland, as he expelled a few puffs of smoke into the hive. "No one knows exactly why, Lelord, but a little smoke is the best way to calm bees."

Sure enough, within a few seconds, the angry buzzing swiftly subsided to a low, peaceful, almost melodic hum. "Sounds like they've forgiven you, Lelord." Mr. Mulholland chuckled. "But from now on, you be more careful. Bees are harmless—friendly,

155

in fact—when you treat 'em right. But if they think you're out
to hurt 'em, they can turn real nasty."

Coming from a man of Mr. Mulholland's reputation, those
were sage words. For Mr. Mulholland was something of a legend
in the community where I grew up. He was reputed to be over
ninety, yet he stood more erect, moved more briskly, than most
men of twenty. His eyes were always clear and twinkling, his
skin smooth and unwrinkled. In a voice that never weakened
or cracked, he loved to talk about his favorite subjects—bees
and honey.

"He comes from a long line of beekeepers," my grandmother
once explained. "You pay attention to every word he says
because, in a whole lifetime, you can't learn all there is to
know about honey."

It wasn't until years later, as a student of the sciences and a
soon-to-be nutritionist, that I appreciated the full significance
of Grandma's advice. In the meantime, I had to be content with
the simple books that Mr. Mulholland gave me to read and with
the homey folk wisdom that he had stored up in his pinpoint
memory.

"Did you know," he once asked me, "that honey may be the
oldest food known to man? Even before they learned to kill
animals, prehistoric cavemen were probably feasting on honey."

"Aw, how do we know that for sure?" I asked skeptically.

"From cave drawings that show men gathering honey from
wild hives. And from earthen pots that archaeologists have dug
up—pots they figure were used to strain and store honey. Far as
they can tell, those pots are at least ten thousand years old,
maybe older."

The earliest religious tracts, Mr. Mulholland went on, attest
to the fact that beekeeping and honey harvesting were performed by every civilization. In the Old Testament is told the
story of how Jonathan, while battling the Philistines, used honey
to restore his strength. St. Ambrose advised his disciples to eat
honey because it "cures wounds and conveys remedies to inward
ulcers." The Koran describes honey as a "medicine for men,"
Muhammad himself having declared it "a remedy for all diseases."

Physicians throughout history had no less a respect for honey.
Hippocrates, the father of modern medicine, wrote, "It causes

heat, cleans sores and ulcers, softens hard ulcers of the lips, heals carbuncles and running sores." Dioscorides prescribed the inhaling of honey for coughs, and he fed it to patients suffering from kidney disorders. Both Galen, the great Greek physician, and Pliny, the Roman naturalist, recommended honey to improve the eyesight.

"You see, Lelord, honey wasn't just a food to these people. They also considered it a medicine."

"Tell me something, Lelord," Mr. Mulholland continued. "Whenever you bruise or cut yourself, what does your grandma tell you to do for it?"

"Rub honey on it," I said.

"Why do you suppose she likes honey better than iodine?"

"Because it doesn't burn, I guess."

"That's one good reason. But there's a more important reason. Honey kills germs, prevents infection."

I was later to learn that honey is indeed an antibacterial agent, because it contains potassium, which creates *hygroscopic power:* the ability to draw off moisture. Deprived of moisture, disease bacteria quickly perish.

Though the ancients had no notion of germs and hygroscopic power, this was no doubt why the Egyptians used honey as a surgical dressing, and the Hindus and Chinese treated smallpox with honey ointments. In both instances, the honey speeded up healing and reduced the amount of scars. Ancient Hebrew physicians prescribed honey for ulcerated wounds, and during the Middle Ages, throughout Europe, honey ointments and plasters—plain or mixed with other substances—were used to treat boils, wounds, burns, and ulcers.

Many Indian tribes of South America still use honey in the healing of wounds and surgical incisions. Slavic farm-folk do likewise with ointments made from honey and white flour or honey and burnt alum. Centuries ago the Norse explorers discovered that the Eskimos of Greenland and Lapland treated burns and wounds with cod-liver oil; Norsemen used honey for the same purpose. The result of combining these different remedies was an ointment, still prevalent in Nordic climes, consisting of honey and cod-liver oil!

As a preventive medicine against all forms of illness and infection, honey is held in high esteem by the tribal peoples of

Africa. When a woman of the Wa-Sania tribe gives birth, her only diet for several days afterward is honey and hot water. For a week after circumcision, the male children of the Wa-Sanias are restricted to the same honey and water mixture. Before circumcision, the Nandi tribesmen place some honey on the child's tongue. As a general medicine, the Nandis mix honey with the bark and leaves of their local vegetation.

But honey's preventive and curative powers don't stop there. It's been used against a vast number of illnesses, many of which were first revealed to me by Mr. Mulholland.

"Take diphtheria," he said to me during another visit. "Do you know that in many parts of the world, it's still a major disease among children?"

And then he told me how European peasant women successfully treated this dread malady by rubbing a chunk of honey deep into the sick ones' throats and air passages. They also applied a honey poultice around the neck, and a few drops of warm honey in the ears, to prevent accompanying pain, ringing, and inflammation.

Though deadly, diphtheria is no longer a major menace; many related illnesses still exist, ranging from the common cold and sore throat to croup, bronchitis, and asthma. In many parts of the world—even in the United States—people still attack these sicknesses with the same folk and kitchen remedies described to me years ago by the wise old beekeeper.

Among opera singers, who must rid themselves of throat infections swiftly and surely, honey remains a favorite remedy. Some prefer it mixed with tincture of benzoin; others like it combined with lemon juice and glycerin. For throats that feel slightly husky, the divas lean toward honey and hot milk. One singer told me that before he goes out to do an aria, he clears his throat by gargling a solution of honey and alum, which is also an old-world recipe for ulcerated gums and mouth.

No matter where my travels take me, I still meet beekeepers who recommend Mr. Mulholland's favorite remedy for the flu: a tablespoon of honey and some lemon juice, dissolved in a glass of hot water. For simple coughs, the beekeeping "fraternity" recommends a mixture of honey, sulfur, and turpentine.

As a respiratory medicine, honey remains very popular among Slavic and Mediterranean farm-folk. These peoples' forefathers were the originators of a bronchitis cure consisting of a tablespoon of honey in a glass of warm milk. Tuberculosis they treat with compounds of honey and buttermilk or goat's milk. For general respiratory conditions, they always keep handy a concoction that includes anise, pepper, horseradish, ginger, mustard, and garlic—all mixed together with honey.

"You're just a little boy now, Lelord"—Mr. Mulholland talking again—"and you sleep like a log every night. But one day, when you're older, something will be bothering you—like a big exam you have to take in school or some kind of business problem when you're on your own. Suddenly, no matter how hard you try, you won't be able to fall asleep, and that'll leave you even more tired and worried in the morning."

"That's called insomnia, right, Mr. Mulholland?" I chimed in proudly.

"You're way ahead of me, son. But did you know that honey is a sure cure for insomnia?" And he told me a number of cures, some of which are still widely practiced.

The Romany Gypsies perhaps came up with the tastiest one. It consists of two tablespoons of honey and the juices of one lemon and one orange squeezed into a tumbler. Just before bedtime, add hot water to the tumbler and drink it down. Not only is this remedy claimed to be more effective than over-the-counter tranquilizers, but it's also more nutritious.

For mild cases of insomnia, the early settlers of the Vermont mountains came up with a simple cure that their descendants still swear by: a tablespoon of honey each night at mealtime. When these people are especially keyed up, they mix three teaspoonfuls of apple cider vinegar in a cupful of honey. At bedtime they swallow two teaspoonfuls of the mixture and, if they are still awake an hour later, two teaspoonfuls more. Because they don't have to worry about overdosing, they can repeat the procedure at hourly intervals, until sleep comes. Old Vermonters will tell you, however, that two, maybe three "doses" are all you'll ever need in one night.

As a soporific (sleep inducer), honey is still widely prescribed by European naturopaths and by conventional physicians, too. Some recommend a tablespoonful or two by itself. Others prefer it mixed with lemon juice and hot milk or water. Natives of Scotland prefer a remedy handed down by their Highland forefathers—pure heather-honey.

Chinese medicine, which combines ancient folk wisdom with

modern science, prescribes, for insomnia, honey mixed with chopped ginseng and dried orange peel. The patient swallows it just before bedtime.

What makes honey such a versatile medicinal food? As I learned from Mr. Mulholland, the answer starts with bees, who manufacture it in their hives from flower nectars, which they gather daily. Flowers provide the bees' final product, honey, with an abundance of two natural sugars, dextrose and levulose, which are predigested. That means, instead of fermenting in your stomach as ordinary cane sugar does, dextrose and levulose are quickly absorbed into the bloodstream, with a minimum of strain on your digestive tract.

It also means that honey, with its 1600 calories to the pound, is the second greatest energy builder, surpassed only by dates, which have a slightly higher calorie count. Honey contains six times the fuel value of milk and an even higher fuel value than meat, fish, poultry, eggs, grains, and vegetables.

The nectar that bees bring to the hive is also mixed with pollen from the plants. Pollen, being rich in nutriments, thus provides honey with such vital vitamins as thiamine, riboflavin, ascorbic acid, pyridoxine, pantothenic acid, and nicotinic acid. Depending on the amount of pollen that the bees consume, the quantity of these vitamins varies with each jar of honey.

Amino acids, the great protein builders, are found in honey, as are the following healthful acids: acetic, citric, formic, malic, and succinic. Besides dextrose and levulose, honey contains, in much smaller quantities, other rare sugars, among them sucrose, dextrine, and maltose. In honey are found the enzymes catalase, diastase, inulase, and invertase—all aids to digestion and assimilation.

Honey also contains minute amounts of iron, copper, silica, manganese, chlorine, calcium, potassium, sodium, phosphorus, sulfur, aluminum, and magnesium. Compared to refined sugar, which has been stripped of all nutritional value, these trace elements make honey a significant blood-builder when used as an everyday sweetener.

Referring to honey in the treatment of anemia, Dr. H. A. Schuette of the University of Wisconsin declared, "The hemoglobin which we build from our food has the power of carrying oxygen to the tissues of our bodies. Without iron content, hemoglobin would not have the power of holding oxygen. Copper has the power to unlock the therapeutic quality of iron in restoring the hemoglobin content of the blood of patients afflicted with anemia."

Because of its energy-building properties, honey has been used in the treatment of weak hearts since time immemorial. Dr. G. N. W. Thomas is among the many contemporary physicians who have rediscovered honey's use in this connection. In an article in the British medical journal *Lancet,* Dr. Thomas described the case of a pneumonia patient who was rapidly sinking as his heart gave out. Heart and pulsebeat were returned to normal with two pounds of honey, prompting Dr. Thomas to conclude that "honey should be given for general physical repair and, above all, for heart failure."

Centuries ago the folk healers of ancient China already recognized this fact. To stimulate blood circulation, they prescribed a mixture of honey, cinnamon, and ginseng potion.

In the years that Mr. Mulholland extolled honey's virtues to me, diabetes was a dread disease, afflicting greater and greater numbers of victims. "You know what's causing that to happen?" the old beekeeper said angrily one day. "White sugar. If the sugar refineries ever succeed in pushing us honey suppliers out of business, they'll also succeed in creating a nation of diabetics!"

Those were strong words, especially since Mr. Mulholland didn't have the "scientific" training to mouth them with authority. Not till many years later did I appreciate their prophetic significance. That was in 1929 when Dr. F. G. Banting, the discoverer of insulin, stated, "In the United States, the incidence of diabetes has increased proportionately with the per capita consumption of cane sugar. In the heating and recrystallization of the natural cane sugar, something is altered which leaves the refined product a dangerous foodstuff." Other authorities have issued similar warnings.

Insulin, of course, must be administered to patients suffering extreme diabetes. But how many of them would have reached that stage, had they consumed honey instead of refined sugar? Science has not yet come up with an answer to that question, but certain facts are indisputable. Before the discovery of insulin, homeopathic physicians successfully treated many diabetics with honey, after taking them off sugar. Among the ancients, who consumed large quantities of honey, diabetes was virtually unknown. Even today, among "primitive" people who haven't been exposed to the sugar-laden foods of modern civilization, diabetes rarely occurs.

The Indians of Northern Mexico learned this lesson the hard way. As their consumption of honey slowly gave way to refined sugar, cases of diabetes increased. Tribal medicine men, sensing the connection, took their patients off sugar and fed them large quantities of honey dissolved in tea brewed from the leaves of the manzanilla plant. In all but extreme cases, the diabetic symptoms vanished or decreased markedly.

Because of its sedative and mild laxative properties, honey has always been a favored treatment and preventive for children suffering from sleeplessness and constipation. At the same time, its hygroscopic properties make it an excellent cure for an age-old problem—bed-wetting.

The Vermont mountaineers treat this childhood problem with a teaspoon of honey at bedtime. Not only does the honey calm an overactive nervous system (a frequent cause of bed-wetting), it also attracts and holds fluids, thereby taking a load off the kidneys and bladder. By lessening bedtime fear and tension in the child, this remedy invariably leads him to self-bladder control, at which time the treatment can be suspended.

In Ireland many mothers still cling to the old Gaelic belief that honey is the best all-around tonic for their children. Bedouin Arabs continue to raise their young ones on a mixture of honey and buttermilk. Honey with cream or butter is used by many peoples to protect adolescents against tuberculosis, while honey and barley water are used as a laxative. In primitive tribes, where worms remain a prevalent problem in children, honey is an important ingredient of many cures.

As a remedy and even a cure for ulcers, beekeepers all over the world recommend honey. This, too, harkens back to antiquity, when many of the great physicians praised the virtues of honey as a medicine for all intestinal ailments.

Scientific research continues to find justification for this aspect of honey's curative powers. Its ability to destroy bacteria was long ago proven. Because it is predigested, it doesn't remain in the stomach long enough to cause fermentation, a condition that not only aggravates ulcers but also attracts disease germs. In fact, in *any* sickness that demands minimum strain on the digestive tract, honey is the easiest, most soothing form of nutrition.

Centuries ago there existed an old wives' tale that bee-stings cured rheumatism. But in recent years this ancient "superstition" was shown in the laboratory to have much merit. For honey contains some of the neutralizing acids found in bee-venom—acids that militate not only against arthritic and rheumatic pains but also against muscular atrophy, numerous nervous conditions, and tubercular glands. An old Hungarian cure for a gouty toe is to wrap it in a honey poultice; this relieves the pain within a couple of hours.

Through the ages honey-drinks took numerous forms, each with its own reputed therapies. *Hydromel,* a mixture of honey and water, was described by Pliny, the great Roman historian, as an invigorator and a cure for fever. *Oxymel,* consisting of honey, vinegar, sea salt, and rainwater, was used for centuries in the treatment of sciatica, gout, and rheumatic ailments. *Oenomel,* a combination of honey and unfermented grape juice, was long used in the treatment of gout and numerous nervous disorders. Many modern honey remedies resemble these concoctions of the ancients.

The quality of honey varies according to the flowers from which the bees extracted the pollen and nectar, the condition of the soil in which the flowers grow, and the prevailing climate. How well I remember Mr. Mulholland peering up at a sky that had been overcast for days, and commenting, "Without rain or sunlight to nourish the plants, my bees won't be bringing us as good a batch of honey."

But however high the quality, many people believed that honey worked best as a medicine when chewed in the combs where the bees stored it. Comb honey is honey in its raw form, still sealed in the tiny, airtight compartments of beeswax.

Science is still analyzing the composition of beeswax, in an attempt to learn what makes it particularly effective against nose and throat ailments, and against allergies like asthma and hay fever. One theory is that, in addition to the components of the nectar and honey, the wax combs contain a greater quantity of raw pollen.

When a person suffers from hay fever, doctors treat this allergy by injecting extracts from the pollen of the plants to which the patient is allergic, until the patient develops immunity. In a similar fashion, immunity is built up by chewing pollen-laden honeycaps (sealed combs of honey). Describing an experiment with Army personnel suffering from hay fever, Dr. George D. McGrew of the Army Medical Corps declared, "Among the many home remedies for the treatment of hay fever, one alone seemed of great value. Several individuals stated that in the past year or two, they had received varying degrees of relief by eating honey produced in their vicinity, and particularly from the chewing of the honeycomb wax."

The honeycomb is also a widespread kitchen remedy for sinus trouble. This discomforting, often painful condition results from an inflammation of one or more of the eight sinus cavities in the head. The inflammation is accompanied by excessive alkaline-urine reaction in the body's chemistry. For some reason which is still not clear to scientists, the chewing of honeycaps brings relief by shifting the urine reaction from alkaline to acid.

POLLEN

Plant pollen, which the bees carry back to their hives and store as food, has itself been an age-old folk medicine. It is mentioned in the Bible, the Koran, and the Talmud, as well as in ancient writings of China, Greece, Russia, and Persia. Hippocrates and other physicians prescribed it to ward off the afflictions of aging.

Raw unstrained honey was one of mankind's first supertonics because it contained the largest amount of pollen. In ancient Greece, where the Olympic Games originated, athletes-in-training were fed large quantities of pollen-laden honey because of the extra energy it provided.

Mr. Mulholland used to gather pollen by scraping the bottom of his hives. He explained that he learned this technique from the Russian peasants, who had to eat the scrapings because they were too poor to keep the honey in their hives. They were forced to sell it.

"The Russians didn't know it"—he laughed—"but that was a blessing in disguise. Scrap from the hives is almost pure pollen, which may be even healthier than the honey."

"Then why," I asked, "aren't people eating more pollen?"

"Because there isn't enough to go around. And that's a shame, Lelord, because there's as much pollen in the world as there are grains of sand, but we haven't found an easy, inexpensive way to gather it."

Which proves that Mr. Mulholland didn't know everything! Some years later I uncovered a Chinese method of pollen gathering which is still used. It consists of fishing the lakes and waterways with specially constructed cloth nets. After being strained, the pollen that remains is left to dry. Then all foreign matter is removed, and the pollen is crushed down to a powder, which is finally sealed and stored in clay containers.

It is said that the Chinese survived famines by consuming cakes made from pollen and honey. Arabs, who had to travel for days through the barren desert, made similar use of pollen gathered from date trees.

Pollen always stirs in me a regretful memory. Many years ago, while collecting data among the Sinitic mountain tribes of Laos, I came upon a most incredible folk-treatment. A native woman was applying globs of pollen, bound into an ointment by honey and royal jelly, to her breasts. When I asked why, my guide explained that one of the breasts contained a lumpy mass—to me, a symptom of tumor! The woman also ate large quantities of pure pollen throughout the day.

Why do I call this a "regretful" memory? Because, at the time, I considered the treatment farfetched, unworthy of serious speculation. I had all but forgotten the experience until 1948, when a U.S. government report described encouraging results on mammary tumors and other cancers in mice treated with pollen. Since then, I often wish that I'd stayed longer in the Laotian hills to observe the outcome of pollen treatment on the native woman and others like her.

A similar pollen-honey-royal jelly ointment is used by the Chams of Cambodia to shrink hemorrhoids, cure all skin diseases, and heal wounds. When a Cham tribesman feels approaching symptoms of gastric ulcer or chronic bronchitis, he gets near-instant relief from a few mouthfuls of stored pollen grains.

Among the thousands of pollen-eating peoples I visited, I was struck by one clear fact: There was not a single case of hay fever, asthma, or other respiratory allergies. At first glance this seems like a paradox, since so many allergies are caused by pollen.

But experiments in Sweden, France, and the United States have shown that patients can be immunized by controlled injections or oral doses of the very pollens to which they're allergic. Without realizing it, natives who eat pollen have probably inherited centuries of immunity to ailments that still plague "civilized" lands!

Pollen's tonic and blood-building properties are recognized by all the natives who gather and store it. Among the Karens of Burma, mothers add extra pollen to the diets of children who appear underweight or anemic. Hill tribesmen of Thailand set aside special crocks of pollen for their elderly, who eat extra quantities to preserve their vigor and virility. Women of the Burmese Shans keep their skins moist and wrinkle-free with an ointment made from pollen and honey.

In the dense Malaysian jungle can be found one of the most fascinating pollen remedies. There, throughout many tribes, pollen is the basis of treatment for nervous and psychological problems. Combined with local herbs—either as powder or cake —it is taken by natives to relieve depression or anxiety, raise morale, and decrease irritability. Usually within a week the patient returns to a feeling of calm and well-being. Mixed with other herbs, pollen becomes a cure for insomnia, as well.

The medicinal value of pollen was dramatically illustrated by the experience of a pilot shot down by the Japanese during World War II. In the Japanese prison camp, his weight dropped from one hundred and seventy-five to eighty-five pounds in one year. Finally unable to work, the pilot was scheduled for execution. To discourage him from attempting an escape, the Japanese seared his feet with red-hot irons.

But the pilot decided to take his chances, and that night he fled the camp. Eluding capture, he was forced to move slowly because of the agonizing burns on his feet. His only diet was berries and shoots. Before long the wounds on his feet developed gangrene. Hopelessly exhausted, the pilot finally lost consciousness.

When he awoke, he found himself in the hands of a friendly Chinese jungle tribe. After bathing him and cleaning the dead flesh from his feet, the tribesmen applied a thick coat of pollen to his feet, followed by a layer of warm honey. Reed bandages held the dressings in place.

In a matter of days the gangrene vanished and the pain was gone. Nurtured on meals consisting of pollen with fruits, herb tea, and broth, which were later expanded to include honey, pollen cakes, fish, vegetables, and meat, the pilot was back on his feet in three weeks.

The pilot, Lieutenant Colonel Thomas J. Tretheway, later described the physical condition of his rescuers. They were tall and had lean bodies and perfect teeth. There were no noticeable illnesses even among the most aged. Pollen-honey cakes were a staple of their diet, and powdered pollen was stored as medicine.

Natives in the jungles of Burma and neighboring Cambodia eat and store pollen in similar fashion. Excavators of the ancient Temple of Angkor Vat, in Cambodia, discovered that pollen was an ancient folk remedy for sexual impotence in the male. This belief still prevails among the natives.

Modern laboratory findings have lent a great deal of credence to that centuries-old "superstition." For pollen contains all the nutrients needed for proper functioning of the prostate, the gland that controls erection and ejaculation. An ailing, enlarged prostate can cause sexual difficulties ranging from complete impotence to premature or painful ejaculation. It is also responsible for internal bleeding and urinary blockage.

In recent years Swedish and German urologists have been experimenting with pure pollen as a medicine for prostate troubles. The results have been extremely encouraging. In many cases, ailing prostate glands were brought back to normal size and function, with all urinary and sexual problems eliminated.

Now gathered by more sophisticated techniques, and available in tablet form, pollen has become one of the most updated folk medicines. Herbalists, naturopaths, and many orthodox physicians are taking the lead from the jungle tribesmen who, for centuries, have used it as a cure for such diverse ailments as rickets, anemia, weight loss, enteritis, colitis, blood poisoning, and constipation.

ROYAL JELLY

In the legends of tribal Africa appear a number of references to a rare, amber-colored jelly that was extracted from beehives. Far less abundant than honey, it was hoarded and distributed only to privileged members of the tribes—the chiefs and the wisemen. This substance was believed to contain a "life-force" that not only cured all illness but also preserved youthfulness.

The Toltec storytellers of Central Mexico sing the praises of a sweet-sour tasting substance from the hive that turned white hair to black, made food easier to eat, restored sight to failing eyes, made the hands stop trembling and the bones stop aching. Chieftains fed it to their wives to preserve their charm and beauty.

History is replete with similar tales of a "youth elixir" produced by the bees, but it wasn't until 1792 that this unique food got its present name, royal jelly. By that time, naturalists had noted that royal jelly is the only food eaten by the queen bee.

Later studies revealed that royal jelly is a glandular secretion of the worker bees. It is fed to bee larvae for the first three days after hatching, but only the queen larvae remain on this "royalty" diet. The remaining bees switch to pollen and honey for sustenance.

And therein lies the legendary mystery of royal jelly. For the queen bee matures more rapidly and grows to nearly twice the weight and size of the workers. And while the ordinary honeybee lives for forty days, the queen can remain alive for as long as eight years, laying twice her weight in eggs daily.

Though steeped in magic and mysticism, the ancients' high regard for royal jelly has been bolstered by recent analyses, which show that this food contains many of the nutrients associated with longer-lasting youth. In France and Mexico, it is even now being prescribed by physicians as a remedy for chronic diseases of the aging—like arthritis and rheumatism—to make, in the words of the Toltec storytellers, "the bones stop aching."

To many tribal descendants of the Mayans in Guatemala royal jelly is strictly a medicine. Never eaten as mere food, because of its rarity, this beehive product is rationed by tribal healers as a cure for infected tonsils, nose and throat infections, and respiratory disorders. It is also fed to aged tribesmen who show symptoms of arthritis, rheumatism, and hardening of the arteries.

Nomadic African tribes hoard royal jelly as both a tonic for the aged and a body builder for the young. It is eaten by men and women on long treks whose bones start to ache, and by infants learning to walk. Together with honey, royal jelly is used by tribesmen as a salve to heal deep wounds and prevent infection.

German scientists, analyzing royal jelly, found it tremendously rich in pantothenic acid, biotin, and nucleic acid. Deficiency of pantathenic acid causes a beefy, furrowed tongue, premature gray hair, and painful, burning feet. As many neuritis and in-digestion victims have benefited from this vitamin, so too have they benefited from royal jelly. A deficiency of biotin is known to bring on conditions associated with aging.

Dr. Thomas S. Gardner also found pyridoxine or vitamin B_6 present in royal jelly. Having a soothing or sedative effect on the nerves, this vitamin aids in easing Parkinson's disease, the trembling palsy so often seen in older people.

Perhaps this was the illness the Toltecs meant when they told how royal jelly "made the hands stop trembling." The biotin and pantothenic acid may indeed have accounted, in some mea-sure, for the extended youth and charm of the chieftains' women.

And if royal jelly actually "made food easier to eat" for the Toltecs, that's because it contains many of the twenty known amino acids, broken down by the bees into their most digestible forms, to be more completely assimilated by the young bees. Scientists therefore feel that persons who cannot utilize many protein foods can assimilate the proteins of royal jelly.

Whether eaten in the form of honey, pollen, or royal jelly, the products of the modern beehive have, under the scrutiny of modern science, more than justified the claims made for them by the ancient folk healers, herbalists, and physicians. Many of their reputed cures still sound like exaggerations, but the number grows smaller as the laboratories continue to break down the intricate mysteries of all three substances. This is what my grand-mother must have meant when she said, "In a whole lifetime, you can't learn all there is to know about honey."

HONEY REMEDIES FROM AROUND THE WORLD

Asthma

> ½ onion
> 2 cloves of garlic
> 1 pint Irish moss jelly
> ½ cup honey

Combine onion, garlic cloves, and Irish moss jelly, and simmer for half an hour. Let cool and strain the mixture through a sieve. Add the honey to a pint of the strained mixture.

Take one tablespoon every two hours, sipped slowly. Alternate with honey alone or honey mixed with water and lemon juice.

An Old Indian Recipe

> 1 egg
> lemon juice
> honey

Place the egg in a wineglass and cover with lemon juice. Leave for twelve hours, to soften the shell. Remove shell and beat yolk and white together. Add honey equal to the amount of lemon juice used. Bring mixture to a boil, and when it starts to get thick, remove from the stove. Bottle it when it cools.

Dose: One teaspoonful, night and morning.

Coughs

Folk Medicine—From Vermont

> 1 lemon
> 2 tablespoons glycerine
> honey

Boil the lemon slowly for ten minutes. This softens the lemon so that more juice can be gotten from it. Cut the lemon in half and extract the juice with a lemon squeezer. Put juice in an ordinary drinking glass. Add glycerine. Stir glycerine and lemon juice well, then fill up the glass with honey. Apple cider vinegar may be substituted for the lemon juice. Regulate the dosage according to your needs, one teaspoonful at a time. As the cough gets better, lessen the number of times you take it. This syrup does not upset the stomach and can be taken by children as well as adults.

Coughs, Hoarseness, and Whooping Cough

> 1 pound onions
> 2 ounces honey
> ¾ pound brown sugar
> 2 pints water

Peel and chop onions finely. Combine honey, onions, and brown sugar with the water and simmer gently over low heat for three hours. When the mixture is cool, bottle and cork it well.

Treatment is four to six tablespoonfuls a day.

Hypertension

Take the juice of half a fresh lemon with a tablespoonful of honey diluted in a tumbler of warm water everyday. This will help steady nerves and bring normal sleep. It is also good for throat infections.

Indolent Ulcers

> 1 ounce yellow wax
> 4 ounces honey

Melt the wax and slowly add the honey, stirring well. Apply twice a day and bandage.

**Abscesses, Boils,
and Skin Ulcers**

Honey-Fig Poultice—From Arabia

Slice a ripe fig in half, dip the cut side in honey and bind it to the affected area. Change the poultice two or three times a day, or as often as necessary until the drawing stops and healing is well under way.

Modern experiments have proved what the ancients knew instinctively: Honey destroys harmful bacteria and promotes healing. And the drawing power of figs was recorded by them long ago in this proverb:

> "Fig-poultice will our bodies rid of tumors,
> Scrofula, boils, and even peccant humors . . ."

Honey Green Surgical Dressing—From Switzerland

This chlorophyll-rich healing poultice should be made fresh each time, and the amount used depends upon the size of the area treated, so exact measurements are not given.

Combine pulped comfrey leaves with enough honey to make a spreadable mixture. To each tablespoonful of the honey-comfrey mixture, add one small garlic clove, finely chopped. Mix well. Spread on a piece of fresh cabbage leaf cut just large enough to cover the infected area and bind in place. Replace with a fresh dressing as the drawing, healing, and antiseptic powers of the remedy extract the inflammation and impurities from the wound or infected area.

**Insect Bites
and Stings**

Honey-Soda Healer—From Ireland

Mix honey and bicarbonate of soda to form a consistency that will adhere to the skin like a salve. Cover the injury with a thick coat of the mixture and allow to dry. (If you are treating a sting, be sure to remove all of the stinger first.)

Honey-Eyebright Lotion—From England

A combination of honey and the herb called eyebright is an old European remedy for eye ailments, from weak, inflamed, and bloodshot eyes to conjunctivitis and ulcers. Honey, with its antibacterial and healing properties, is also said to strengthen the eye tissues, and eyebright lives up to its name in promoting the health and strength of the eyes.

Culpeper once said of this eye-strengthening herb, ". . . If eyebright were as much used as it is neglected, it would have spoilt the trade of the spectacle-makers."

¾ pint boiling water
1 handful eyebright, flowers and leaves
3 tablespoons honey

Pour the boiling water over the eyebright, cover, and let stand until lukewarm. Strain. Add the honey and stir until dissolved. Soak cotton pads in the lotion and place over the eyes, leaving the pads on fifteen to twenty minutes, adding more lotion as needed to keep them moist. The eyes may also be bathed with the lotion several times a day.

Honey-Milk Eyebright Lotion—From Scotland

The Scots have a similar eye lotion, made the same as the English version except that they substitute ¾ pint of milk for the boiling water.

Honey Herbal Gargle—From Egypt

For sore throat and as a refreshing mouthwash.

2 tablespoons honey
½ pint sage tea
½ pint cider vinegar
1 teaspoon oil of sweet almonds
5 drops oil of cloves

Dissolve the honey in the hot tea and stir in the remaining ingredients. Bottle and use as needed.

**Insomnia and
Nocturnal Leg
Cramps**

Honey-Buttermilk Nightcap—From Spain

> 2 tablespoons honey
> 1 glass buttermilk
> Juice of 1 lemon
> White jasmine flowers (optional)

Dissolve the honey in the buttermilk and stir in the lemon juice, mixing well. The relaxing properties of honey and buttermilk make them an ideal sleep-inducer, the easily assimilated calcium in buttermilk helps prevent leg cramps, and lemon has so many medicinal values that it can benefit almost any minor ailment that's keeping you awake. In Andalusia, Spain, I was served this drink topped with white jasmine flowers, not to add to the remedy, but for their aesthetic value.

Honey-Barley Strengthening Gruel—From India

This combination is an old folk remedy valued for its strengthening properties, its healing effect on the internal organs, as a remedy for blood disorders and a general rundown condition, as a nerve tonic and invigorator, and for its nutritive benefits, especially for invalids and infants.

Its blood-cooling factors make it a favorite of East Indians and Arabs.

> 4 ounces whole barley
> 1½ pints water
> 3 ounces honey
> Peel of 1 lemon, well washed

First bring the barley to boil in just enough water to cover, and strain off. Pour the 1½ pints of water over the cleaned barley, and simmer gently until the barley is soft, adding more water to keep it at 1½ pints as it boils away. Remove from the fire and stir in the honey. For a thinner honey-barley liquid instead of a gruel, add more water during the cooking until the desired consistency is reached.

Honey-Sunflower Iron Cordial—From Quebec

¾ cup sunflower seeds
6 cups water
1 cup chopped dates
½ cup raisins
1 small orange, washed and quartered
1 piece ginger root, about 4 inches long
1 cup honey

Place the sunflower seeds in a saucepan; add the water and all other ingredients except honey. Bring to a boil, reduce heat, and simmer gently about thirty minutes.

Remove from the fire and let steep until lukewarm. Strain. Stir in honey, mixing until it dissolves.

Dose: A wineglassful once or twice a day, or as needed for energy.

Clogged Arteries
and High Cholesterol
Artery-Conditioning Tonic—From Germany

2 teaspoons honey
1 tablespoon lecithin granules
2 teaspoons safflower oil
1 cup fenugreek tea

Dissolve the first three ingredients in a cup of fenugreek tea, stirring well. *Dose:* one cupful a day as a preventive, and two or more as a remedy if the arteries are already clogged with cholesterol deposits. May be drunk either hot or cold, but because of the oil I find it more palatable to drink hot.

Honey acts as a natural tension-reducer; safflower oil provides the polyunsaturated fats necessary to balance the intake of animal fats; fenugreek tea contains small amounts of two fat-emulsifying vitamins, choline and inositol; and lecithin is rich in both of these artery-conditioning ingredients, plus many more.

(For the many excellent honey cough and cold remedies, see Chapter 6.)

13

Lactic Acid: The Fountain of Friendly Bacteria

In the quiet hours of evening, you could hear it fermenting in my grandmother's cellar. Sometimes the expanding "brew" would seep out, sending a delightful, near-intoxicating aroma through the house.

Grandma was very thorough. During the first week or so, she visited the cellar several times a day, to remove surface scum from each crock, while her trained nose sniffed out the degree of fermentation. The end result was one of the most delicious and, as I was later to learn, one of the most healthful foods known to man: sauerkraut.

How come? As a first step to learning the answer, take a quick inventory of your state of health. Do you have frequent headaches and stiff joints? Are you troubled by bouts with insomnia, postnasal drip, constipation, stuffed sinuses? Perhaps, like the frantic actresses on TV commercials, you repel people with bad breath, body odor, dried-out hair or blemished, yellow skin. Are your eyes listless and easily strained, your weary muscles easily fatigued? In general, do you feel "all washed-out"?

If you answered "yes" too often, then it's time for you to make the acquaintance of one of man's best friends. This creature neither walks nor talks. You can't teach it to perform tricks or to obey commands. It's so tiny, in fact, that you can see it only under a microscope. It goes by the unlikely name of *Lactobacillus acidophilus,* and its job is to supply the body with one of the most potent nutrients folk medicine has contributed to science— *lactic acid.*

Though you can't feel or hear the roar of gunfire, your body is a battleground for a war that's taking place every moment of your life. One of the combatants is your old friend *Lactobacillus acidophilus.* Its enemy is a vast spectrum of putrefactive bacteria that are trying to conquer your body. The enemy's chief "headquarters" is your large intestine—the bowel—but it also inhabits other parts of your digestive tract.

The enemy bacteria produce poisonous substances that circulate through your bloodstream, clogging every cell in your body. Unable to ingest a proper supply of food and oxygen, and to dispose of wastes in a normal manner, the cell loses its vitality, its ability to grow, even its ability to reproduce. Multiply this cell-sickness by the billions of cells in your body, and you'll begin to understand where many of your physical troubles begin.

By feeding the "good guys"—the bacteria that destroy the toxic organisms—lactic acid helps to keep your cells healthy and vigorous. Consumed in the form of sauerkraut and other fermented foods, it performs myriad functions to keep *you* healthy and vigorous late into life. It may even prolong your life by as much as ten, twenty, even thirty years.

Small wonder that in Germany, where sauerkraut is practically a dietary staple, it's put to many medicinal folk uses. Bavarian villagers always keep a jar of the juice handy, to relieve attacks of dyspepsia. In the hills overlooking the Rhine, mothers feed their children sauerkraut snacks as a cure for skin ailments and tooth decay. An old Alsatian laxative combines sauerkraut juice with tomato juice or honey.

As folk medicine, lactic acid dates back to pre-Biblical times. Sauerkraut is only one of the numerous foods in which this nutriment is present. Far more widespread, as food and folk medicine, is the spectrum of lactic acid sources known as fermented milk or cultured milk. The most famous of these is yogurt.

Galen, the famous Greek physician of the second century, claimed that yogurt had a beneficial, purifying effect on a bilious stomach. In the seventh century, there was published in Damascus a treatise called *The Great Explanation of the Power of the Elements and Medicine,* in which learned physicians from Greece, Arabia, Persia, Syria, and India recommended yogurt for soothing, refreshing, and regulating the intestinal tract and for "strengthening the stomach."

The French recount an old legend that tells how the ill and aging Emperor Francis I regained his health and strength upon eating a "secret formula" prepared by a man who brought it all the way from Constantinople. The court physicians were so impressed by their emperor's miraculous recovery that they paid thousands of francs for the "secret formula," which turned out to be yogurt. From then on, goes the legend, yogurt became known in France as *lait de lavie éternelle*—milk of long life.

In a section of Yugoslavia, there lives a people whose average life span goes well beyond one hundred years. For most of these years, they remain active, robust, vigorous, and virile. Arthritis and other degenerative diseases are virtually unknown to them. Few suffer from hardening of the arteries or other forms of senility. Fascinated by these people's health and longevity, the great Russian scientist, Professor Elie Metchnikoff, traveled there to investigate their eating habits and living conditions.

What he found, among other things, was a diet rich in lactic acid foods—yogurt, sour milk, black sourdough bread, and sauerkraut. Metchnikoff, who had already theorized that much of the body's health is dependent upon the health of the large intestine, concluded that *Lactobacillus acidophilus* and one of its "cousins," *Lactobacillus Bulgaricus,* played a crucial role in the people's well-being.

"Investigators," he wrote, "have attributed the stability of milk to the presence of certain microbes that hinder the putrefaction of milk. These are, in particular, the microbes that sour milk—that is, cause the formation of lactic acid—and which are antagonistic to the microbes of putrefaction. The lactic acid microbes hinder the multiplication of the organisms of putrefaction."

More recent evidence of lactic acid's versatility comes from the study of another land of hardy centenarians—the natives of Tamish, in the Soviet Republic of Abkhasia. Describing their life-style in her book, *Abkhasia: The Long-Living People of the Caucasus,* Dr. Sula Benet states, "Much of their excess crop is pickled, not canned. In this way, they preserve enzyme values and provide a little lactic acid."

Even among the oldest Abkhasians, Dr. Benet found no evidence of cancer, thus bearing out a study described some time ago in *World Medical News.* According to researchers at the Bulgarian Academy of Sciences, this journal stated, "The harmless, rod-shaped organism which makes yogurt out of milk (and kefir) , *Lactobacillus Bulgaricus,* turns out to have a potent anti-tumor activity. Injections of *Lactobacillus Bulgaricus* extracts, they say, can cure several types of experimental cancers, and appear to be effective against human skin tumors."

One of the foremost studies of lactic acid was conducted by a European researcher, Dr. Johannes Kuhl, who recommended, as protection against cancer, a wholesome, natural diet reinforced with liberal daily amounts of lactic acid fermented foods. Specifically, Dr. Kuhl mentioned sauerkraut, yogurt, buttermilk, clabber or other soured milk, cottage cheese, and such fermented foods as pickled beets and pickled cucumbers.

In many parts of the Caucasus, the natives prefer another lactic acid food, called kefir. The kefir grain, with its fermenting yeasts and bacteria, is added to fresh milk, which is then permitted to sour. Many naturopaths consider kefir the best remedy for digestive troubles, because it breaks up into tiny particles (as compared to yogurt, which holds together or breaks into lumps) .

Armenians of the U.S.S.R. drink extra quantities of kefir to relieve chronic constipation and to stimulate waning appetite. Both Armenians and Georgians for centuries have regarded kefir as medicine for tuberculosis and typhoid. Research has found a far lower incidence of diarrhea among Caucasian infants whose mothers wean them with kefir instead of whole milk.

A complete list of fermented milk remedies would read like a world atlas, with each country contributing its own native variation. In the Chilean Andes, a drink called skuta is taken for diseases of the stomach and liver. Icelanders drink skyr to purify the blood and tone up the body. Chass, a fermented milk from India, is taken as a cure for dysentery.

As a skin-cleanser and beautifier, fermented milk has been treasured by women of all civilizations. Mosab, an ancient Persian product, is still drunk by Iranian women to preserve their youthful complexions. Throughout Scandinavia, females drink tette, a product prepared from boiled milk and the leaves of the tette, a native meadow plant. The hardy Tartar women of the Crimea believe that koumiss—fermented mare's milk—keeps them young, attractive, and vigorous.

Koumiss is fast achieving renown as a remedy for one of mankind's dread diseases. Oriental scientists, investigating native uses of this fermented milk product, have concluded that it's a potent factor in the treatment of tuberculosis. As a result, many koumiss sanatoriums have sprung up throughout the Far East. In other lands, according to the World Health Organization, sanatoriums treat tuberculosis with a milk culture called airig. Though ancient peoples had no knowledge of lactic acid, they certainly responded to its anti-infection properties. Finnish farmers still drink a fermented milk product, called ropa, to ward off pneumonia. Gooddu, a Sardinian variety, is fed to patients suffering from laryngitis and pharyngitis. In Turkestan, the peasants treat ear infections with drops of a lactic acid milk called busa.

Buttermilk, one of the most popular lactic acid drinks, is a traditional folk remedy of the American frontier. On many a farm, its "friendly" intestinal bacteria are still considered the best cure for constipation or diarrhea. When mothers detect the slightest allergy to ordinary milk, they immediately switch their children to buttermilk. If troubled by chronic heartburn or gas, old-time farmers swallow a wineglassful of buttermilk before and after each meal. Ounce for ounce, buttermilk is regarded as the best thirst-quencher when working under the hot sun.

The lactic acid content of sour cream has made this thick fermented milk product a favored external as well as internal folk remedy. Hungarian peasant women, famous for their sour cream sauces and gravies, turn the cream into a cooling salve when treating their children for hives, ringworm, or other rashes. In the Carpathian Mountains of Rumania, farmers treat gastritis attacks by applying cold sour cream poultices to the pained area, then going onto a twenty-four-hour diet of sour cream and cottage cheese (another lactic acid food). Dalmatian grove-tenders in Yugoslavia treat gouty joints with an ointment made from sour cream and olive oil.

When yogurt or cheese ferment, they produce a by-product called whey. Norwegian farmers chew on solid whey, or bathe their mouths with a liquid form, to relieve gingivitis and other inflammations of the gums. Many dentists in Norway prescribe whey for children prone to excessive cavities. Recently, in England, researchers recommended adding whey to ices, as a means of reducing tooth decay.

Once considered commercially useless—except as fertilizer and animal food—most whey wound up in the garbage heaps of modern milk-processing plants. Only lately has science begun to acknowledge whey's potential as a medicinal food. Whey, in powder or tablet form, is sold in health-food stores.

Many other lactic-acid folk remedies have successfully withstood the skeptical scrutiny of science. Dahi, a fermented Indian milk similar to yogurt, kills streptococcus and staphylococcus germs on contact. Salmonella and shigella, two forms of dysentery that plague the Near East, occur rarely among natives who drink leben, a curd culture. Early experiments tend to confirm that oraka, a Palestinian drink, and hangop, a Dutch fermented milk product, are both effective against tension and migraine headaches.

The result of all the ongoing research has been a widespread growth in the use of this folk remedy by modern herbalists and nature healers. Some years ago, while on a lecture tour of Germany, I had occasion to visit the clinic of a well-known naturopath. To all his constipated patients, he served a side salad consisting of uncooked sauerkraut and fresh yogurt. Behind this treatment was the theory that sauerkraut acts as a gentle "broom" to sweep out delayed fecal matter in the bowel, while providing lactic acid to encourage growth of friendly bacteria and to "sweeten" the intestinal tract. The yogurt, too, provided lactic acid and acted as a tonic for the intestinal tract.

If constipation is one of your problems, this natural remedy can be duplicated in your own kitchen. All it takes is a small dish of drained sauerkraut, with a spoonful of yogurt plopped on top. Or if sauerkraut is not your "cup of tea," you might try another old-world recipe for constipation: yogurt mixed with prunes or prune-whip. The bulk provided by any fruit, in fact, complements the stool-softening properties of yogurt.

With the galloping growth of antibiotics in modern society, many doctors have discovered a new application for yogurt. One of the risky side effects of antibiotics is their ability to destroy healthful bacteria in addition to the disease-bearing ones. To counteract this effect, yogurt is prescribed at the same time or immediately afterward, to replace the friendly bacteria destroyed by the chemical remedy.

In addition to repairing the damage done by antibiotics, yogurt performs an antibiotic function of its own. Studies conducted in Turkey, and later in Denmark, found that yogurt is capable of destroying two types of tuberculosis bacilli in humans and another type that strikes cattle.

"Lactic acid milk," said the late Dr. William MacNider, "has saved the lives of more children than diphtheria antitoxin." An eight-ounce jar of yogurt, it was found, has an antibiotic value equal to fourteen units of penicillin.

As a digestive aid, lactic acid had been found to be of great value—especially in the elderly. That, perhaps, is another reason why the Abkhasians not only live long but also retain their youthful vigor. For, as we grow older, our bodies tend to lose their ability to produce an important digestive juice, hydrochloric acid. We may be eating the healthiest of food, but without a proper amount of this bodily chemical, much of the food passes through our intestines improperly digested. Lactic acid, from any source, can substitute, in part at least, for hydrochloric acid to perform the same digestive function.

In buttermilk, yogurt, and other milk sources, the lactic acid combines with another vital health agent, calcium. This mineral, so vital in maintaining the strength of the bones and the heart muscles, also needs hydrochloric acid to be digested. Lactic acid not only pinch-hits as a digestive juice but also combines with calcium to cure one of our commonest ailments—insomnia.

What do you do when you're having a sleepless night? If you have an aversion to barbiturates or other sleeping pills, your answer will probably be "Drink a glass of warm milk." Milk is not bad, but the next time you're battling with insomnia (or if you're a chronic insomniac), try an ancient cure recommended by the long-lived mountain people of Bulgaria—buttermilk.

During the sleep cycle, calcium feeds the nerve-ends which conduct the stimuli from the brain to the nerves, the muscles, and the bloodstream, and then back to the brain. When this cycle is operating efficiently, with lactic acid in the blood sending the calcium forward to the sleep center of the brain, it's impossible for the conscious mind *not* to sleep at regular intervals.

If the bloodstream doesn't contain enough calcium and lactic acid, the operation of the cycle is not efficient. The complex sleep center, which controls our sleeping and waking, cannot produce the drowsiness and inactivity of the conscious mind necessary for sleep.

Another lactic acid food, acidophilus culture, has proved immensely valuable as an antihistamine. By destroying a particular strain of putrefactive bacteria in the intestinal tract, it affords immense relief to persons suffering from ulcers and allergies. These bacteria, which produce histamine—a substance abundant in the blood of allergy sufferers—cannot cope with the friendly bacteria carried by lactic acid.

For persons who are allergic to milk itself—and there are many of them—the fermented variations are almost always successful replacements. Nearly anyone is able to tolerate yogurt or acidophilus milk. Buttermilk, too, makes a fine substitute. Among the farmers of Europe and Asia, allergic infants are fed yogurt prepared from fresh cow's milk or goat milk, beaten until the curds are small. Another efficient lactic acid product is acidulated milk, made by adding lemon juice to fresh milk.

Acidophilus culture, available in many health-food stores, is a unique source of lactic acid—particularly for people who need a fast-acting, powerful, but safe laxative food. It contains the beneficial bacteria in concentrated form, but must be taken with milk because these bacteria need milk sugar (lactose) to survive. If there is an allergy to milk, a tablespoon of the culture and a teaspoonful of milk sugar can be combined with any juice.

Gout patients have derived enormous benefits from acidophilus milk and yogurt. That's because gout results from excess uric acid, and the lactic acid of these foods produces bacteria . that dispose of uric acid in the intestines.

Have you ever taken an oral antibiotic and then found that your skin was turning dry, scaly, itchy? Chances are that the antibiotic was destroying one of the B vitamins, biotin, by killing off the intestinal bacteria that produce it. The concentrated lactic acid in acidophilus culture, or in large amounts of yogurt, quickly remedies this condition. All the B vitamins, in fact, and also vitamin K, can be synthesized by these friendly bacteria.

It is for this reason that bad breath (halitosis) can be remedied by consuming lactic acid foods, because this condition, usually accompanied by stool odor, is often the result of a vitamin B_6 deficiency, caused by putrefactive bacteria in the bowel.

The Balkans enjoy adding various raw vegetables and spices to their sauerkraut. Sliced onions, carrots, and turnips are favorite taste-toppers. So are small green tomatoes, cucumbers, and red peppers—whole—as well as garlic, celery, and cauliflower —chopped. Seed spices, such as caraway, dill, and celery seed, not only add to the flavor but also aid in the fermentation. Instead of salt, try adding, to your seed-spice mixture, kelp seasoning and/or garlic powder, two palate-teasers that are loaded with medicinal value. (See basic recipe at end of chapter.)

Nor do you have to stop there. Among the great joys of sauerkraut is the amount of experimenting you can do with it after it's ready to serve. One of my grandmother's favorite additions was natural cider vinegar. Sesame seeds and sunflower seeds were two mouth-watering garnishes that she also handed down to us.

Cold or warm, sauerkraut can be served with any nonstarchy vegetable that suits your fancy. Only one thing to remember, if you prefer your kraut warmed: It should be cooked over a low flame because overheating can destroy the lactic acid and enzymes it contains.

Shredded cabbage, of course, is the basis of all sauerkraut, but practically anything that grows can be fermented into a lactic acid food. "Sauer" lettuce, kale, and spinach are popular variations all over the world. In the wine country of France, I've savored the natural sweetness of fermented grape leaves, and in the Italian countryside I've been treated to soured escarole flavored with anise. The first time I lectured an Alaskan audience on the values of sauerkraut, they did me one better by introducing me to fermented Eskimo rhubarb, coltsfoot, and purslane. From one of my daughter's young soul food friends, I learned of a Southern variation—fermented collard greens.

Many appetizers, side dishes, and relishes make fine sources of lactic acid. The Jews of Hungary, Rumania, and other Eastern European lands rarely serve a meat dish without the accompaniment of pickled cucumbers and green tomatoes. Pickled or marinated herring are also favorites of the Jews, as well as the Scandinavians. Italian tables are frequently adorned with raw string beans, cauliflower, kidney beans, and red peppers that have been pickled in vinegar. Numerous French meat and fish entrees are served with *sauce marinade* (marinated sauce) or *sauce vinaigrette* (vinegar sauce) .

If you have neither the time nor the inclination to make your own lactic acid foods, you can, of course, purchase the commercially made products. But a few words of caution:

In buying ready-to-eat yogurt to be used for health purposes, stay away from the flavored varieties which are loaded with sugar and coloring matter. Get the *plain* variety. If you have a large family, it may pay you to invest approximately ten dollars for a yogurt maker, which is carried by most health-food stores. For additional information on the uses of yogurt, the reader is advised to get a copy of my comprehensive cookbook, *Cook Right—Live Longer.*

When buying commercially prepared sauerkraut, get the "kosher" or barrel variety, usually sold in *bulk* in Jewish or other ethnic stores. And, of course, the varieties sold in health-food stores are highly recommended because they are free of artificial chemical preservatives, to say nothing of sugar and excess salt with which the average commercial varieties are loaded.

You'll also find an assortment of other lactic acid foods and acidophilus cultures in health-food stores—a type of store that can supply you with so many of the unusual foods not to be found in the average market. Do locate one near you and patronize it regularly.

For those who would like to make their own yogurt and/or sauerkraut, the following basic recipe for each will be of special interest:

YOGURT (basic recipe)

To make the first batch of yogurt, get fresh yogurt *culture* to be used as a starter (available at health-food stores) .

Scald, but do not boil, one quart of fresh milk. When milk cools to 100 degrees, add the yogurt culture starter, mix thoroughly to break up milk solids. Pour into prewarmed, sterilized jars; cover tightly.

Place jars in large pan of warm water. Set pan on a warm radiator, over the pilot light of the kitchen stove, in an unlit oven with only pilot light burning, or use one of the many yogurt makers on the market (all of which have special instructions for best use) .

Leave the "activating yogurt" strictly alone for at least two hours or until it has set to a custardlike consistency. Place in the refrigerator to cool. (To make a thicker yogurt, add 1/3 cup of powdered skim milk for every quart of fresh milk before pouring into glass jars—*stirring thoroughly*.)

Note: You need the yogurt culture as a starter only to make your first quart of yogurt. After that, simply save ¼ cup of your *fresh,* homemade yogurt to use as a "starter" for the next batch, proceeding according to the recipe above.

SAUERKRAUT (basic recipe)

Shred large head of cabbage into earthenware crock (at least 1 gallon capacity). Arrange in layers 1-inch thick. Sprinkle 1 teaspoon sea salt over each 1-inch layer. Repeat layers until crock is filled. Cover with plate weighted with heavy object. Keep in warm place. Next day remove any foam or "scum" that will accumulate at top, *after which* stir cabbage. Do this each day. You may add 1 tablespoon caraway or dill seeds and, if desired, sliced onions, cucumbers, other sliced vegetables. At end of three or four days, after foam or bubbling has stopped, transfer to jars and cover tightly. Store in cool place for use as needed.

14

Water: The Medicine Everyone *Can Afford*

What's the first thing you do when you wake up in the morning? Chances are that you reach for the radio and tune in the weather report. "Bright and sunny," says the forecaster, and you heave a sigh of relief—no trouble deciding what to wear today.

But what happens when you hear "cloudy, chance of rain" or "intermittent showers throughout the day"? Instantly, you're beset with problems. Should you carry an umbrella? Wear a raincoat? Maybe it'll rain so heavily that you'll need rubbers to protect your feet.

To most city dwellers and suburbanites, rain portends trouble and inconvenience, for it means having to guard against getting wet. Even farmers, who welcome precious rain for their crops, bundle up to keep even a single drop from touching their skins.

In some parts of the world, however, rain has just the opposite effect. It is a signal to remove all clothing and drench the body. Many African native tribes believe that pure rainwater is sent by the gods to rid the body of evil spirits. When rain falls in the Amazon jungle, it touches off a rite, among numerous aboriginal tribes, which consists of stripping bare and dancing in the downpour. These Amazonian aborigines believe that rain gives them strength and power.

Primitive superstition? Pagan worship? Perhaps. And yet, in many civilized lands, rain is treated with the same respect, if not the same amount of ritual. German peasants encourage their children to romp naked in the fields during a rainstorm. When summer rains come to France and Scandinavia, farmers stop their chores and take time out to bathe in the water from the sky, exposing as much of their bodies as modesty permits.

Water, plain and unadulterated, has frequently been called the world's cheapest medicine. In an age where this "medicine" is as close as the nearest spigot, it seems hard to believe that water has been used methodically, throughout history, to maintain health and to cure illness.

Hippocrates and his disciples treated innumerable ailments with water that was first boiled and then strained. For general well-being, Hippocrates recommended water in its purest form: rain. In the absence of rainwater, he listed, in order of preference, spring water, well water, snow, and ice.

Tourists today still marvel at one of ancient Rome's legacies—her public baths. As artistically designed as the temples and palaces of that period, Roman baths numbered over a thousand, and one of them was equipped to accommodate twenty thousand patrons at a time. The Greeks and Persians, too, erected mighty, ornate structures to house their public baths.

History records that the Emperor Augustus was cured of a fatal disease with water, when all other remedies failed. Charlemagne, king of the ancient Franks and ruler of the Holy Roman Empire, held court while immersed in a tub of warm water. During the Middle Ages, when an outbreak of leprosy reached epidemic proportions, bathing became a religious duty among the Germans.

Still popular today are the Turkish baths and Finnish saunas, which date back into antiquity. German spas, with their health-giving mineral springs, still thrive as treatment centers for numerous ailments, as do the hot-bath centers of Japan and the steam houses of Russia.

If you find these facts "quaint" and amusing, consider for a moment the composition of your body. A man weighing 150 pounds is almost 75 percent water. About 80 percent of the blood and 75 percent to 80 percent of the muscles are water. The gray matter of the brain consists of about 80 percent water.

All life processes start in water and must be continued in water. Water helps cleanse and flush impurities from the body. To neglect regular water drinking is to leave the body wide open to many infections, some of them fatal. To minimize the value of simple bathing is to clog the pores of your skin with dirt from the outside and poisons from within.

Water, known as the "universal biological solvent," loosens waste matter in the bodily organs and dissolves poisons in the blood. Through the kidneys, lungs, and sweat glands, it eliminates toxic substances and disease bacteria. Without sufficient water, the blood may thicken and circulate poorly.

Hot water expands the blood vessels, cold water contracts them—more safely and speedily than any drug known to science. It is this dual property of water that gives it its unique medicinal value. For just as a bath or shower affects the circulation of the entire body, water applied locally—whether in the form of a spray, dip, or compress—has the same effect on circulation in the part of the body being treated. If you have never tried any of the other folk remedies in this book, you have surely, at one time or other in your life, used plain old water—with the full approval of your physician!

Have you ever had a nosebleed? What did the doctor recommend? Most likely, an ice pack or cold compress, applied to the top of the nose or the back of the neck. Why? Because the sudden cold contracted the vessels in that part of the body, thus reducing the flow of blood there.

How about the time you came up with a sudden cramp in the leg or arm? Did you try the "old-fashioned" remedy of a hot compress on the aching limb? That, too, is what the first-aid manuals prescribe—because the heat expands the vessels, bringing extra blood to nourish and relax the tightened muscle.

These two simple, basic principles—cold contracts, heat expands—form the foundation of water cures all over the world.

Among the peasants of Sicily, a common cure for gas pains is a cold compress on the abdomen. Their neighbors, along the nearby coastline of Italy, attack the same condition with a steady spray of cold water on the hips.

There is no known cure for arthritis, but during a trip through the Congo, I witnessed one of the most dramatic remedies. An aged native lay in the hut of a tribal medicine man, his joints contorted and wracked with pain. Patiently, the medicine man applied hot-water compresses, replacing them frequently, hour after hour. I couldn't believe my eyes when the old man

finally rose to his feet, smiling, opening and closing his fists pain-
lessly, wiggling his toes.

Actually, it shouldn't have come as any surprise to me. I had
long ago learned that arthritis is associated with poor circulation
to the afflicted area. The increased flow of fresh blood probably
eased the arthritic deposits around the old man's joints.

Many folk remedies are as simple as taking a bath. In New
Guinea, when an Arapesh woman is having a difficult pregnancy,
she goes into the shady part of the jungle and immerses the
lower part of her body in a cold stream until the discomfort
vanishes. To ease the discomforts of menstruation, Arapesh
women perform the same act in a vat of water heated to the high-
est bearable temperature.

By trial and error, people all over the world have discovered
the varying effects of hot or cold baths on a wide range of ailments. For centuries the peasants of Uzbekistan have treated gas
pains by simply immersing the lower half of the body in a cold
tub. To ease backaches, they do the same in a tub of hot water.
The relaxing properties of the hot half-bath are also a remedy
for constipation, while the contracting effects of the cold half-
bath ease the symptoms of hemorrhoids.

These forms of partial bathing, common among all cultures
since the dawn of civilization, eventually gravitated to still another ancient remedy that is used widely in hospitals and sanatoriums everywhere. It is called the sitz bath and is prescribed
by physicians for a wide variety of ailments. *"Sitz"* is the German
word for "sit," and as its name implies, the sitz bath is a bath for
the rectal and genitourinary areas, which is taken in the sitting
position.

Taken hot, the sitz is an effective pain reliever for patients
suffering from inflammation of the bladder, uterus, ovaries, and
vagina. It is also used to bring on delayed menstruation and to
relieve pains in the hips.

A cold sitz has an inhibiting effect on the menstrual flow and
is therefore recommended to control excessive bleeding. Sim-
ilarly, it is prescribed as a control for hemorrhaging of the
bowel, uterus, and vagina. Blood discharge, caused by an ailing
kidney or bladder, is often checked, too.

Sitz tubs can be purchased in medical supply houses and in
most well-stocked drugstores. Built to fit snugly over the rim of

the toilet bowl, they provide the most comfortable method of taking a sitz. Or you can innovate your own tub at home.

German farmers keep a large vat handy for first-aid sitz baths. The vat must be large enough to accommodate the user's pelvic region, and shallow enough for him to rest his feet comfortably on the floor. In the absence of any small tubs or vats, the ordinary bathtub makes a workable substitute when filled just high enough to cover the patient's hips.

For patients suffering from excessive fatigue and decreased vitality, European naturopathic clinics have devised a unique application of the sitz bath: alternating hot and cold water. The patient sits in the hot unit for about fifteen minutes, then immediately shifts to a cold tub for about thirty seconds. This is done alternately, three or four times in succession.

In a hot sitz, the temperature ranges from 105 degrees to 110 degrees. Temperatures from 50 degrees to 60 degrees constitute a cold sitz. The neutral (warm) temperature range is from 85 degrees to 95 degrees. The same temperature distinctions apply to ordinary baths as well.

And make no mistake about a plain old "ordinary" bath. Besides cleaning the skin, it has had many uses as a folk remedy. In every land, soaking the body in a hot tub is a standard method of relieving fatigued or sore muscles. When a child in rural France is struck by scarlet fever, the mother immediately places him in a hot bath, to bring out the rash. The residents of Provence use the same treatment to bring out the rash of measles. Throughout all the Balkan countries, chronic rheumatism is relieved by a ten-minute hot bath, taken just before bedtime.

Because a full-body bath in water of neutral temperature relaxes the blood vessels of the skin, it tends to draw excess blood away from the brain and spinal cord. It also has a soothing effect on nerve endings in the skin. That's why the Berbers of Libya, for centuries, have regarded the neutral bath as a relief for nervousness and excessive irritability. The Maoris of New Zealand immerse themselves in neutral waters as a remedy for hives and other skin irritations. When curing alcoholics, many Slavic people use the time-tested method of their forefathers to ease the symptoms of withdrawal—a bath in warm water every three hours.

As for cold bathing, "It prevents abundance of diseases. It promotes perspiration, helps the circulation of the blood, and prevents the catching of cold." This was an opinion written in 1776 by John Wesley, the founder of the Methodist Church, who devoted much of his life to the study of folk medicine.

As a remedy for fever, regardless of the ailment, the cold bath is a worldwide household remedy. The Helvetii tribes of ancient Switzerland used to cure mild depression with an ice-cold bath. Tibetan mountain-dwellers take daily cold baths for all manner of respiratory illnesses, ranging from the common cold to pneumonia. Ear, nose, and throat infections are treated in the same manner.

Among the Eskimo Indians of northwestern Canada, such "civilized" diseases as measles, German measles, and chicken pox were unheard of until European explorers touched their shores. Later came the white missionaries, bearing religion and science. To their Eskimo beneficiaries, these three relatively mild illnesses proved extremely debilitating, if not fatal, because their bodies contained none of the necessary antibodies to fight the disease germs. Against such odds, the white man's medicines were next to useless.

According to their legends, the Indians were visited one day by a medicine man who said he had been dispatched by their gods. He ordered them to forswear the white man's "poisons" and, instead, to soak their bodies in ice-cold water, six times between each sunrise, whenever these diseases struck. The Indians followed these instructions and, if legends are to be believed, astounded the missionaries with their swift recoveries. Though their bodies are now more accustomed and inured to the once-deadly ailments, these Eskimo Indians still use the cold bath treatment prescribed by the wise old medicine man.

Earlier I mentioned that the Provençals treat measles with *hot* baths. Is the Eskimo treatment a contradiction? Not at all: It merely demonstrates the unique versatility of cold water as a cure. That's because the net final result of cold bathing is heat.

To understand this biological process, think back to the last time your ears or your fingers were exposed to freezing temperatures. First there was pain, then numbness, which lasted until you stepped into the warm indoors. Remember what happened then? Within a few minutes, the numb parts of your body turned red-hot, almost as if they were feverish.

And therein lies the "secret" of cold water remedies, even where heat is the recommended treatment. The initial effect of the cold is to contract the blood vessels, to close the pores, to cause a chilling sensation of the skin, to irritate the muscles connected to hair follicles, causing gooseflesh. But once dry and moved to a warm environment, the patient experiences an opposite reaction, as the vessels dilate and blood rushes back to counteract the cold, opening the pores to release perspiration and to warm the chilled skin and muscles. In other words, the end product of cold bathing is relaxing, comforting warmth!

Cold water over the body, whether in the form of bath or shower, is considered by many folk cultures to be the best all-around external tonic. By tightening the skin, it retards wrinkles and produces a natural color that's far safer than the artificial effects of drying pancake makeup. It stimulates the blood, the muscles, the nerves, and the glands, thus increasing hormone production. By stimulating the metabolism, it improves digestion.

Native island dwellers and coastal inhabitants derive an extra benefit from their water cures: sea salt. Besides remedying ailments with heat and cold, saltwater provides many healthful minerals that are absorbed through the skin. Farmers of the British Isles, who live too far inland to reap the benefits of seawater, create their own homemade baths with packaged sea salt —about five pounds per tubful.

In the mountains lining the Mexican shores live many Indian tribes. They have added an unusual variation to standard water cures. Near the surf, they dig a hole large enough to accommodate the patient's body and deep enough to allow seepage of water from below. They then cover the patient with sun-heated sand, leaving only his face exposed, and pour saltwater over the sand until it cakes. The patient remains in this sand pack for about a half hour, his skin slowly soaking up the minerals from the sea. This treatment, say the Indians, relieves the symptoms of rheumatism and arthritis, purifies the blood, relaxes a strained nervous system, and soothes digestive disorders.

Spraying with a jet of water is another folk remedy that's widespread. As a cure for the common cold, the nomad Pathans, of Afghanistan, fill a goatskin bag with hot water, then shoot it out through a narrow nozzle, directing the stream all over the patient's body. If, however, the cold is complicated by bronchial congestion, they alternate the jet sprays with hot and cold water. The Tephus of Bhutan relieve muscle tension with a sharp jet of hot water directed at the cramped area. For headaches and eye-strain, they direct a cold stream of water at the forehead. The spray has the added advantage of combining massage with the water treatment.

Though primitive peoples must devise unique methods of creating a jet stream, we "moderns" need nothing more than a garden hose or adjustable shower-head. More sophisticated applications of ancient water treatments can be found in the Finnish saunas, in the vapor baths of Russia, and the hot-air baths of Turkey. Americans consider steam bathing a great way to relax and lose weight, but this thousand-year-old tradition has far greater applications in the countries of its origin.

Steam is created by throwing water over hot stones. Subjected to temperatures as high as 200 degrees, the body's glands and organs are stimulated, while most bacterial and viral growth are retarded. This, in turn, enables the body to wage a stronger fight against disease.

But, by far, the greatest advantage of steam bathing is the elimination of bodily wastes and poisons. At that temperature, the sweat glands are stimulated into increased activity and the pores of the skin open wide. Out flows the perspiration, containing uric acid and other substances that normally emerge from the kidneys in the form of urine. For persons whose kidneys and bladder are not functioning at peak capacity, this in itself is a tremendous boon. The excessive sweating takes a load off those eliminating organs of healthy people, possibly extending their lives.

The Finns, in their saunas, add an extra step. After the steam treatment, they dive into a cold pool or lake, or, in the winter-time, they simply go outside and roll in the snow! Then they return for another dose of heat in the sauna, soap themselves with warm water, and finish off with a dash of cold water over the entire body.

So far I've confined this survey of water remedies to bathing principles. But what about the *drinking* of water? As a necessary means of maintaining healthy nutrition, balanced blood, and clean, functioning organs, water is taken for granted. Just to stay healthy, the body needs from six to eight glassfuls a day. But can water also be classified as a curative agent?

Throughout the world—but especially in Europe—exist sites of an age-old health tradition—the mineral spring. Long before European conquerors touched the American shores, Mexican Indians were treating their sick and aging with mineral waters and natural hot-spring waters. Where hotels, clinics, and rest homes now stand in Saratoga Springs, New York, Indian shamans once relied on the mineral-rich waters that still bubble forth there. Ancient Arab physicians pinpointed desert oases whose unique waters had curative properties. Maps of Russia and Germany are virtually pockmarked with spas to which people have journeyed for centuries—and still do.

These spas, approved of and supervised by the government, not only offer mineral water for bathing and drinking, but also for inhalation, irrigation, and douching. Under the supervision of doctors, patients are treated for numerous ailments under a total program of diet, rest, bathing, and drinking.

Arthritis, for example, is treated by placing the patient on a fast and feeding him nothing but the natural waters. Elderly people return to spas frequently, to take treatments for high or low blood pressure, weak hearts, and circulatory disorders. The water cure, as it is called, has been successfully used, for two thousand years, in the treatment of such diverse conditions as blood diseases, nervous disorders, chronic inflammation of the organs, eczema, allergies, and hormonal disorders.

In an experiment on American hospital patients, researchers concluded that mineral waters play a significant role in reducing the blood-cholesterol level. Research in Hungary has demonstrated that mineral water strengthens connective tissue and increases the body's natural immunity to disease. The same researchers also found that spa treatments for arthritis were far more effective than doses of cortisone. In Russia, where immunology holds a high rank in the scientific disciplines, the Academy of Sciences recommends spas as the best places to build up the body's natural defenses against disease.

Water cures throughout history have ranged from the sublime (walking barefoot in the dew) to the ridiculous (as a cure for mental illness, Wesley prescribed holding the patient under a waterfall!) . Some are as easy to find as the kitchen sink; others require long trips to faraway places.

However you come by it, water is the least costly, most plentiful folk remedy in the world. Of course, it can't be regarded as a cure-all, but there's not a physician alive who'd question the wisdom of frequent bathing or the age-old stricture for whatever does or doesn't ail you: *Drink plenty of water.*

15

Fenugreek: An Ancient Solution for Modern Pollution

What are you doing to protect yourself against the pollution of your body's vital organs? Most people, upon hearing this question, reply with remedies they take for the nose, throat, and lungs—the respiratory area, where we breathe pollution.

Few of us are aware that pollution can be swallowed as well as inhaled, thereby striking at the kidneys, the bladder, the liver, and the entire intestinal tract. It can even damage the heart and the reproductive organs. And modern science, with all its synthetic chemicals and "wonder" drugs, has yet to come up with a safe protection against bodily pollution.

Though they couldn't have known it at the time, it was the ancient inhabitants of Asia and the Mediterranean shores who first discovered an antipollutant for the body. It was the marvelous herb called fenugreek, a word derived from the Latin term *"foenum Graecum,"* meaning "Greek hay." Eating it first for its tasty flavor, these peoples were quick to recognize fenugreek's efficacy in reducing fever, soothing inflamed stomachs and intestines, easing women of the pains of abscess, ulcer, or stoppage of the uterus.

For centuries, in the tiny Asian principality of Bhutan, Lepcha tribesmen have made unique use of fenugreek as a preventive and cure for blood poisoning. After moistening the seeds ever so slightly, they grind them down to a thick paste. The paste is then applied as a poultice to deep gashes, boils, chancres, ulcerations, and other skin conditions.

In neighboring Tibet, natives brew the roots, stalks, and seeds of fenugreek into a strong decoction, which is then added to a small mugful of boiled milk. When the mixture cools, it is drunk as a medicine for constipation and irritation of the bowel.

But what have these treatments got to do with pollution? To understand how fenugreek combats, soothes, and sometimes heals such afflictions—and how this all ties in with the poisons we eat or breathe—it is important first to understand one of your body's chief functions.

Each time you cough or blow your nose, you are ridding yourself of a substance known as mucus. Most people, especially those who are prone to colds or allergies, accept mucus as an everyday fact of life—which it is. What few of us realize is that mucus is not confined to the nose and throat; it exists in many of our vital organs and throughout the intestinal tract.

A certain amount of mucus secretion is healthy. In its natural, liquid, free-flowing state, mucus serves as a cleanser and lubricant. However, if mucus becomes thick, stale and stringy, difficult to eliminate, it can be a danger—and therein lie the hazards of pollution.

Compare your body to the engine of an automobile. Every driver who lives in a dust-ridden or smoke-filled area knows the inevitable result: sludge. Oil, grease, and other lubricants become thick and hard. Instead of preforming their lubricating and cleaning functions, they cake on the engine parts and gather filth. If not removed in time, they can clog the carburetor, the valves, the pistons, even the air and oil filters that protect against sludge. When enough sludge accumulates, the engine must break down.

In this respect, the human "machine" is no different from the one that drives your car. Virtually with every breath of air, you are inhaling dust and fumes that mix with the mucus in your system. When you smoke a cigarette or eat a food saturated with chemical preservatives, you further thicken the mucus. The end result is what I refer to as "body sludge."

Unfortunately, coughing, sneezing, and a running nose are not sufficient escape hatches for all of the body's excess mucus. Much of it is deposited in the stomach, and from there it circulates to the intestines and kidneys. Thickened and hardened by pollutants, the sludgy mucus turns stale, slimy, and stringy. Its viscosity becomes sluggish. Unable to flow freely, it turns sticky and starts to pile up instead of passing out through normal body openings.

But this is only the beginning. When excess mucus clings to the stomach and intestinal linings, these linings secrete more mucus to relieve the irritation, thus creating an even thicker mass. Because this excess mucus impedes normal secretion of digestive juices through the stomach and intestinal walls, undigested food particles cling to the mucus mass, further thickening it and forming gas as they start to ferment.

Do you suffer from sour-tasting mouth and bad breath? Do you get frequent gas pains that are relieved only by excessive belching? Perhaps you have more serious afflictions, like ulcers or kidney disease, colitis or even tumors. If so, there's a good chance that your body is riddled with excess, hardened mucus.

It is saturating your cells with a thick, sticky, ropey substance that denies them oxygen and nourishment. It is causing the blood and other bodily fluids to become thick and sluggish. Unable to circulate freely, the blood cannot do a proper job of carrying away waste matter from the cells. Eventually, the cells may become contaminated.

Meanwhile, a similar process may be occurring in your small intestine, where many millions of small glands extract the nutritive elements from digested foods and pass them on to the bloodstream. When these glands, called villi, become clogged with stale mucus, they cannot perform this function at full efficiency; this results in a denial of nutrients to cells throughout the entire body.

Digestion is not confined to the intestinal tract alone. It begins in your mouth, where the first bite of food stimulates the salivary glands into action. The saliva they secrete contains powerful enzymes that begin the digestion of starch and sugar. If the salivary glands become clogged with mucus, they cannot function at optimal speed, and your food will be swallowed partially undigested.

In other words, you may be on the world's healthiest diet and yet be suffering from malnutrition. Which is why no dietary program is complete unless it includes fenugreek. For unless vitamins, minerals, and other nutrients can be digested and

enter the bloodstream, they cannot possibly do the human body
their maximum amount of good. Merely taking them into the
mouth and letting them drop down the throat does not mean
that these vital elements are going to find their way into the
bloodstream. First they must pass through the villi in the small
intestine. And if these villi are heavily coated with mucus, how
in the world are the full concentrations to reach the bloodstream?

In all probability, it was the farmers of ancient Egyptian and
Greco-Roman times who first uncovered the potentials of
fenugreek. By adding its sickle-shaped pods to the fodder of
horses and livestock, they noticed a marked decline in the
animals' secretion of excess mucus. This observation, no doubt,
prompted them to add fenugreek to their own diets, with the
same pleasing result.

Throughout China, fenugreek tea is still a household remedy
for congestion of the nose and throat. The Alfuros of Indonesia,
at the first signs of chest congestion, chew large quantities of
fenugreek seeds, to bring up phlegm. To unstuff the ears and
other cavities where mucus can accumulate, Nepalese Gurkhas
dip their noses into a strong decoction of fenugreek, inhale
deeply, then throw their heads back, allowing the medicine to
circulate freely.

Though their connection with mucus remained unclear for
many centuries, other ailments soon fell prey to the healing and
curative properties of fenugreek. Before long, medical and
paramedical practitioners added this aromatic herb to their
pharmacopoeia as a rejuvenant and restorative.

Nicholas Culpeper, in the seventeenth century, was the first
of the European herbalists to make note of fenugreek's potency
as an aphrodisiac, demulcent, diuretic, nutritive, tonic, and
carminative for stomach gas. But it remained for a priest, Father
Sebastian Kneipp of Bavaria, to bring this plant to full prom-
inence in Europe. Himself a prominent researcher, Father
Kneipp first recommended fenugreek as a gargle, then as a
soothing agent for irritated tissues, and finally as a "liquid
mucus solvent."

All but lost in the modern morass of patent drug remedies,
fenugreek remained forgotten for a time, except to herbalists
and naturopaths, and to veterinarians, here and abroad, who

continued to prescribe it as a remedy for animal ills. In recent years, however, the public had been rediscovering the medicinal and nutritive properties of fenugreek, as it continues to gain greater and greater acceptance.

In the parts of the world where this herb was first discovered, it has never lost its popularity as a food and folk remedy. Indians, who use the seeds as flavoring in chutney and curry recipes, also eat fenugreek to prevent pellagra and numerous nerve disorders. Physicians throughout the Far East and Middle East prescribe it for cases of difficult labor in pregnant women. Iraqi women drink the tea and use it also as a douche for vaginal irritations caused by catarrh (excess mucus).

As a sex rejuvenator, fenugreek is still in widespread use—especially among Turkish women, who eat a mixture of powdered fenugreek and honey, to improve their femininity and sexiness. Men consider it to have a beneficial effect on their sex organs.

Modern science would like to relegate fenugreek's sex rejuvenation powers to the scrap heap of folklore and superstition, but there is evidence to back up this claim. Many men who suffer from sexual impotence or sexual underactivity have been found lacking in vitamin A, and laboratory analysis has shown fenugreek to contain an oil resembling cod-liver oil, which is rich in vitamins A and D.

Another substance found in fenugreek is trimethylamine, which acts as a sex hormone in frogs, causing them to molt and prepare for mating. Diluted solutions of this substance increase flower production in plants. Its effects on man are still in the testing stage.

Analysis made by Chicago's famous Laboratory of Vitamin Technology revealed that 8 ounces of a tea made from fenugreek seeds contained on an average: 45.2 micrograms of thiamine (vitamin B-1), 74.5 micrograms of riboflavin (vitamin B-2), 410 micrograms of niacin, 266 micrograms of pantothenic acid, in addition to even more substantial amounts of choline. While the vitamin content revealed by this test could hardly be termed "nutritionally consequential," still it did prove that a tea made of fenugreek is very definitely a food, especially if used as a pleasant mealtime and between-meal beverage.

Dr. Mohammed El Shahat of Fuad I University in Cairo,

Egypt, extracted a new vitamin from the oil of fenugreek seeds. This vitamin, according to Dr. El Shahat's clinical tests, enabled 345 Egyptian mothers to provide more and better milk for their nursing babies. The new vitamin has been tentatively called H for its human lactation-promoting factor. Small doses of it, found in fenugreek seeds, increased the mothers' milk anywhere from 160 percent to 900 percent soon after the babies' birth. In addition, the quality of the mothers' milk was much better, since it contained greater amounts of proteins, fat, sugar, minerals, and vitamins, resulting in healthier, better-nourished infants.

The choline in fenugreek has a particularly vital function. When the liver is not working properly, it deposits fats—lipids, they are called—within its cells, thereby lessening its own ability to perform efficiently. Choline is a valuable lipotropic (fat-dissolving) factor. Even after a single meal with high fat content, choline has been observed to exert its fat-dissolving influence upon the liver.

In a similar manner, choline dissolves fatty accumulations that might occur in the kidneys, impairing their function. And because of its ability to remove accumulations of fat (cholesterol) on the arterial walls, which causes these blood vessels to lose their elasticity and to harden, choline is used widely by today's heart specialists in the treatment of arteriosclerosis.

But most vital of all is the mucus-cleansing power of fenugreek. Just as "flushing oil" dissolves hardened accumulations of oil and grease in your car engine, so too does fenugreek tea soften and dissolve hardened masses of accumulated mucus.

That's because fenugreek seeds, when moistened, become slightly mucilaginous (sticky) themselves. In the same way that it takes one oil to dissolve another oil or grease, it takes one mucilaginous substance (fenugreek) to dissolve another more sticky substance (mucus) in your body. The fenugreek solution then remains in your system to form a soothing, protective coating over inflamed, irritated areas, as many an ulcer patient can attest.

Besides dissolving fat in the kidneys, fenugreek can perform its other vital function there. The delicate tubes which make up our kidneys may become congested with mucus. Should that happen, the kidneys—which really are nothing more or less than a filtering plant—cannot perform their normal task of eliminating waste liquids. Pains develop in the back, waste fluids back up into the blood, and the entire body becomes poisoned. Death may result, since uremic poisoning follows a complete breakdown of the kidneys, bringing about stoppage of all body functions.

Between the kidneys and the bladder are a pair of tubes that can become clogged with mucus—the ureters. Whenever you have a bad cold, you may experience the result of this congestion, for the body secretes excess mucus during a cold—mucus that winds up in the ureters. Until the cold is gone, the patient feels a frequent need to urinate, even though smaller amounts of urine are passing from the kidneys to the bladder.

In extreme cases, the curing of the cold is not sufficient to unclog the ureters. Mucus may continue to pile up. To avoid this condition, Armenian mountain folk drink a daily quart of fenugreek tea, not only at the start of a cold but for at least a week after the cold's symptoms have vanished. Armenian city dwellers use fenugreek as medicine for the organs of taste and smell. Before each meal, they down a "cocktail" of the tea, believing that it stimulates these two vital senses.

Actually, they too are deriving the benefits of fenugreek's mucus-cleansing power. For when mucus coats your tongue, clogging the grooves where your taste buds reside, you're likely to be losing much of the enjoyment of food. When too much mucus accumulates around the olfactory nerves in your nose, your sense of smell is impaired. In both cases, a steady diet of fenugreek tea can unclog those vital areas, restoring the senses to normal.

Perhaps the most dramatic demonstration of fenugreek is yet to come. Science has established that there are two forms of anemia: primary anemia, which is the result of an insufficient number of red blood cells, and secondary anemia, which results from hemorrhaging, cancer, weakening discharges, or poisoning. Because secondary anemia weakens the red cells, these cells form a mucus coating, then clump together in masses of sludge.

Not only does this sludge prevent vital tissue cells from receiving adequate nutrients, but it also causes tissue starvation by blocking the entrances to tiny capillaries. Sludged blood can become tightly packed, forming large plugs that settle in the blood vessels. If one of these plugs is jarred loose, it can easily be carried to one of the main arteries, stuffing it up and sometimes causing instant death.

Because of fenugreek's ability to remove mucus from the body, common health sense would indicate its use by any person who has good reason to believe that a certain disease or certain bodily conditions may have caused a mucus coating to form on the red blood cells, thereby slowing down blood circulation to the point where blocks of tissue cells are starving for want of oxygen and nutritive elements. Anyone who is not strictly up to par—either mentally or physically—may suspect that this is exactly what is happening: Sludged blood has so clogged his bloodstream that certain muscles or certain organs become more and more deficient every day, until finally they deteriorate to the point of serious disease.

Whatever the health benefits derived from fenugreek, it also contributes a delightful side effect. Turkish women drink the tea not only to make themselves more alluring to the eye but also to sweeten the breath and body odor.

Scientifically, this makes perfect sense. For unlike soap, toothpaste, and mouthwash, fenugreek cleans the body from the inside. With the intestinal passages, organs, and bloodstream cleared of excess mucus and other poisons, their unpleasant odors are no longer carried by the breath and perspiration.

So potent, in fact, are the volatile oils in the herb fenugreek, and so thorough a job of penetration do they accomplish, that often a delicate fragrance of the fenugreek seeds will emanate from the body pores of a person using the herb regularly as a tea. These oils seek out and penetrate most remote crevices and creases of the membranous linings of the body cavities where unwanted mucus often collects in excess amounts. The oils are also absorbed into the tissues, while some of them finally find their way into the sweat glands.

Fenugreek tea is easily brewed by adding two level teaspoonfuls of the seeds to a cup of boiling water. After allowing it to steep for five minutes, stir it vigorously, then strain it into another cup or wait for the seeds to resettle. Honey makes a good sweetener, and lemon or lime juice adds to its piquancy.

Practically no one today can fully avoid the hazards of pollution, and it will take many years for science to solve the problem completely. In the meantime, don't you owe it to yourself to keep your bodily "engine" clean, in smooth working order? And what better way to do so than with nature's own marvelous cleanser—fenugreek.

16

All the Comforts of Comfrey and Chamomile

COMFREY, THE HEALING HERB

Comfrey, one of the more valuable plants known to botanic medicine, is believed to have originated in the Caucasus Mountains of southern Russia, was imported to England, and soon began to grow both wild and under cultivation throughout most of Europe.

Today its fame as a folk remedy and the cultivation of the plant have spread to many parts of the world, including Australia, New Zealand, Canada, and the United States, where it now grows wild in some states and is cultivated in others.

The powers of comfrey are summed up in three folk names it has acquired over the centuries—*knitbone, knitback,* and *healing herb.*

The earliest recorded claims for comfrey were made by the Greek physician and botanist Dioscorides, and by Pliny, a Roman naturalist and author. Centuries before modern scientific methods isolated the factor that we now know is responsible for comfrey's rare healing power, Dioscorides listed the plant for its wound-healing and bone-knitting properties.

Pliny also praised the wound-healing properties of comfrey, though he was more enthusiastic than scientific when he wrote, "The roots are so glutinative that they will solder or glue together flesh that is chopt in pieces . . . The same [roots] bruised and applied in the manner of a plaster doth heal all fresh and green wounds."

Comfrey's medical properties are listed in various herbals as demulcent, emollient, mucilaginous, pectoral, expectorant, styptic, nutritive, and vulnerary. The first three properties have a beneficial effect on internal and external ulcers and inflamed tissues of the stomach, throat, and other parts of the body. Its pectoral and expectorant factors combine with them to make a powerful remedy for coughs, bronchitis, and other chest complaints.

"Vulnerary" is a name given by ancient herbalists to plants that were used to cure battle wounds. Comfrey's success as a wound-healer has been confirmed through centuries of use.

The earliest recorded comfrey remedies were made only of the root. By the seventeenth century the leaves were being used to some extent, but even then Culpeper wrote, "A decoction of the leaves hereof is available to all purposes, though not as effectual as the roots."

Greeks, Romans, Turks, Saracens, Russians, and Britons used external applications of bruised or scraped comfrey root for wounds, skin ulcerations, boils, and other infections, inflammations, and swellings. The root, boiled in water, was drunk for "all inward hurts."

Broken bones were treated by applying the scraped root on a piece of leather and binding it firmly around the injury, to hold the bones in place until they could knit back together. At a time when doctors who set broken bones were scarce, comfrey aided the healing process so rapidly and consistently that it was given the name of *knitbone*.

For rheumatism and other pains in the joints the same scraped root poultices were applied. Old-timers held leather poultices and bandages in high esteem. Today's poultice of cloth or gauze is just as effective and certainly more sterile.

In some countries, comfrey leaves were eaten in salads or cooked as greens by country folk, or, as one British writer put it, "by those of unrefined taste." Today, even people with "refined taste" eat the tender young leaves of this nutritious plant, make chlorophyll-rich beverages of them in a blender, and drink comfrey tea. For they now know that the leaves are not only high in food value, but they also possess the same healing agent as the roots.

This agent, called allantoin, is described by scientists as "a nitrogenous, crystalline substance which is a cell proliferant." In everyday language, that means it increases the speed at which nature can heal fractured bones, wounds, burns, inflamed tissues, and gastric and duodenal ulcers. Which just about covers what the ancients claimed for it. Wrote one British editor, in *Chemist and Druggist:*

> Allantoin is a fresh instance of the good judgment of our rustics. Comfrey never had a very prominent place in professional practice; but our herbalists were loud in its praise, and the country culler of simples held it almost infallible as a remedy for both external and internal wounds, bruises and ulcers, for phlegm, for spitting of blood, ruptures, hemorrhoids, etc. For ulcers of the stomach and liver, especially, it was regarded as of sovereign virtue. It is precisely for such complaints as these that allantoin is now prescribed.

COMFREY REMEDIES, OLD AND NEW

Comfrey root remedies date back almost to antiquity, but herbalists of those early years omitted any reference to one of the easiest and most pleasant ways of using the leaves, either fresh or dried. If the ancients drank comfrey tea they kept remarkably quiet about it (except perhaps for an occasional slurp).

Only during this century has comfrey tea become one of the best-selling herbal beverages, enjoyed for its flavor and valued for its healthful benefits. Just how beneficial its effects can be is told, in part, by Dr. Charles J. Macalister, the scientist who isolated allantoin from comfrey.

In his book with the short, catchy title of *Narrative of An Investigation Concerning An Ancient Medicinal Remedy and Its Modern Utilities,* Dr. Macalister tells how a bleeding gastric ulcer was cured by drinking comfrey tea. The case was reported to him by a physician in Lancashire, England, who said he was called to see a girl suffering "with gastric ulcer, hematemesis and severe vomiting."

After treating the patient in what the doctor said was "the usual orthodox manner," within three weeks she was well enough to return to her job at the mill. The patient's mother later told him, "Doctor, my girl never took a drop of your medicine, and all she has sipped is pints of strong comfrey tea."

The doctor concluded his report by saying that he had since found comfrey tea to be an excellent sedative for the gastric mucous membrane. And later experiments have shown that comfrey is just as beneficial to duodenal ulcers involving the small intestines as they are to those of the stomach.

German farmers, for centuries, have been drinking strong infusions of comfrey leaves, several times a day, as a cure for kidney stones. Rural Frenchmen take the same treatment for gallstones and minor liver ailments.

Comfrey root poultices have long been a favored folk remedy for gout, but the easy, modern method is to make a paste of water and comfrey root powder and apply it as a poultice to the painful area.

A gout remedy that recently originated in England is said to be effective in reducing pain and inflammation. It consists of soaking the foot in a basin of strong, cool comfrey tea. And while you're about it you might as well soak both feet, to ease aching arches, burning, and plain everyday tiredness.

Asthma is a difficult ailment to remedy, but H. E. Kirschner, M.D., author of *Nature's Healing Grasses,* tells the case history of a farmer in Cambridge, New Zealand, who cured his asthma by eating fresh comfrey leaves. The man had suffered from asthma nearly all of his life until one day he absentmindedly nibbled a comfrey leaf. That night, for the first time in years, he enjoyed a restful, unbroken sleep.

"He decided it must be the comfrey leaf he had eaten," said Dr. Kirschner. "Now he eats some every day, and has not been troubled with asthma since."

If the story concerned just one isolated case, it wouldn't prove much. But other asthma sufferers heard of the "cure," tried it, and they, too, obtained relief. It wasn't long before supplies of comfrey leaves were being shipped all over New Zealand, not only to asthma patients but to those wanting relief from ulcers, digestive disorders, painful joints, and other ailments that comfrey has a record of relieving.

If asthma is a tricky ailment to treat, arthritis in its various forms is even more so. Switzerland's Dr. Alfred Vogel makes no claims for a cure, but he reports that for years the Swiss people have used comfrey as a poultice to relieve the pains of arthritis.

"Externally, one can apply pulped comfrey root to the painful parts," he said, "and you will find that the pain will gradually fade out."

According to Dr. Vogel, the Swiss people have successfully used comfrey for four of the complaints mentioned earlier—ulcers, wounds that refuse to heal, and leg and other external ulcers. He lists the fourth one with this strong endorsement, "There is hardly a better remedy to be found [than comfrey] for the external treatment of gout."

The ancients knew the value of scraped comfrey root for burns, and we now know that the pulped leaves, much easier to prepare, contain the same major healing factor, allantoin. Let's go back to Liverpool, England, 1911, and see how for the first time this healing agent won the support of the medical profession on a wide scale. The report is from Dr. R. W. Murray, Hon. Surgeon, Liverpool Hospital:

> Towards the end of last year, there was an explosion at a factory, and we were called upon to treat a large number of men who were severely burnt on the head, forearms, and face. The burns were mostly of the second and third degree . . .
>
> Dr. Macalister asked me to try dressing them with *allantoin,* and kindly provided us with a quantity of it . . . The results were so satisfactory and so convincing to house surgeons, nurses, and dressers that dressing with allantoin solution soon became general. It not only stimulates epithelial growth, but "cleans up" sloughing surfaces in a remarkable fashion.

The ancients recommended comfrey for all diseases of the lungs, including consumption.

By the time the fifth edition of *Potter's Cyclopedia of Botanical Drugs* was published, both the leaves and roots of comfrey were being used in remedies:

> *Parts used:* Roots and Leaves . . . Comfrey is very highly esteemed as a remedy in all pulmonary complaints . . . wherever a mucilaginous medicine is required, this may be given. A decoction is made by boiling one-half to one ounce of crushed root in one pint of water or milk. Dose, a wineglassful. The leaves are preferably taken as an infusion prepared in the usual manner. Comfrey leaves subdue every kind of inflammatory swelling when used as a fomentation.

Euell Gibbons, an authority on healthful herbs, gives more specific directions for the same remedy, brought up to date, by advising that it be simmered, preferably in milk, in the top of a double boiler for thirty minutes.

Ancient herbalists recommended the external application of scraped comfrey root for hemorrhoids. Most moderns favor the easy method of buying the powdered roots or leaves and mixing the powder with water to form a paste or with vaseline (petroleum jelly) for an instant ointment.

Gibbons suggests an internal remedy based on the one adapted from *Potter's Cyclopedia.* "With ½ ounce of witch hazel leaves added to the milk-comfrey mixture before cooking," he says, "the remedy, taken internally, is said to be a great help for hemorrhoids."

In addition to their healing properties, comfrey leaves contain an abundance of vitamins and minerals. The entire plant is a good source of vegetable protein, and the green leaves contain vitamins A, C, E and several B vitamins, including choline, the fat-emulsifying vitamin that helps fight cholesterol deposits. Other ingredients are folic acid, the antianemia vitamin, and some B-12, which controls the deadly pernicious anemia.

The leaves also contain such vital minerals as calcium, potassium, phosphorus, some iron, a little iodine, and many other trace minerals. Comfrey is one of the richest sources of silicon in the botanic world, surpassed only by horsetail grass. A lack of silicon is found in patients suffering from hernia and ulcers.

If you live where fresh comfrey leaves are available and own a blender or liquefier, you can make a vitalizing chlorophyll-rich cocktail or originate one of your own with whatever greens are handy. All leafy greens contain chlorophyll, and according to a deduction made in 1913 by a German chemist, Dr. Richard Willstätter, "All life energy comes from the sun, and green plants alone possess the secret of how to capture this solar energy."

No conscientious person would tout comfrey or any other herb as being a cure for "every ill of mankind," but comfrey comes closer to it than most. It has such a long and successful record of healing so many diverse ailments that I am in complete agreement with Euell Gibbons' appraisal of it, and I heartily endorse this recommendation by him:

> I am beginning to think that comfrey may have some antibiotic activity that has hitherto been unsuspected. I highly recommend

that those scientists who are now searching for antibiotics in higher plants take a long, hard look at both the leaves and the roots of common comfrey.

CHAMOMILE, THE COMFORTING HERB

Since the days of Dioscorides, chamomile (or camomile) has been used as a calmative in nervous disorders and hysteria, and as a preventive or cure for failing appetite, indigestion, flatulence, and other types of stomach distress. It has also been a relaxing remedy for headache, fatigue, insomnia, and many female complaints, including menstrual cramps and the pains of childbirth.

Old-time herbalists were enthusiastic and often poetic in their praise of chamomile. Gerard prescribed it "for those who are weary to the point of exhaustion" and called it "a plant of great benevolence."

"Chamomile is under the dominion of the Sun," wrote Culpeper, "and of course is good for the stomach, and grateful." He recommended it as a tonic for general debility and to strengthen the stomach, claiming that a decoction of the flowers "taketh away all pains and stitches in the side."

Chamomile contains nerve-soothing calcium in an easily absorbed form, plus a volatile oil and glucoside with specific relaxing properties. These ingredients alone are enough to justify many of the claims made for it.

But the ancients didn't have to analyze chamomile's ingredients to be aware of its contribution to their store of folk remedies. They learned from experience what its healing values were. In Saxony, it was cultivated on a large scale for medicinal use, and in the sixteenth century this condensation of a verse was written in praise of it, using its charming old Saxon name of *maythen* (from a Greek word meaning "earth-apples") :

> "Have a mind thou, maythen,
> What thou accomplishedst . . .
> That never for flying ill
> Fatally fell man
> Since we to him maythen
> For medicine mixed up."

—Saxon MS. Herbal (Harleian) 1585

Maythen, or chamomile, has long since proved its worth "for medicine mixed up." In France and Spain, chamomile tea is a popular after-dinner beverage to prevent or relieve digestive distress caused by overeating. Many physicians, in both countries, still recommend a cup of it at bedtime for insomnia, two or three cups a day as a tonic to lessen some of the discomforts and debility of the aged, and a few spoonfuls with milk as a remedy for colicky babies and children with upset stomachs.

In Spain, chamomile is known as manzilla (little apple) or manzanilla, and if you prefer wine to tea, you can get it in that form, too. The Spanish flavor one of their light sherries, called Manzanilla, with chamomile. This wine is reported to have tonic properties, along with its relaxing and sometimes exhilarating effects.

Hungarian Gypsies make an excellent tonic by adding one-fourth cup of a strong decoction of dried buckbean (or bogbean) leaves to three-fourths cup of chamomile tea. They gather the fresh flowers and leaves in season, dry them, and use the chamomile flowers for tea and in other remedies. From the buckbean leaves, they make a potent medicinal extract, which is used to treat numerous ailments.

For a general rundown condition and all bronchial and lung complaints, including tuberculosis, a favorite Gypsy remedy is a strong decoction of chamomile tea, comfrey root, and elm bark. The dose is half a cup of the decoction mixed with half a cup of hot milk, sweetened with honey.

A popular herbal of the seventeenth century advised the *smelling* of chamomile flowers, not for physical ailments, but as a do-it-yourself tranquilizer that's worth trying:

> "To comfort the brain, smell camomile, eat sage . . . wash measurably, sleep reasonably, delight to hear melody and singing."
>
> —*Ram's Little Dodoen,* 1606

More than a century and a half later, Britain's Sir John Hill was so impressed with the many uses of chamomile that he wrote, "All parts of this excellent plant are full of virtue."

The relaxing, gently healing properties of chamomile have given it the reputation of being "man's physician," but another of its virtues caused it to be known as "the plant's physician."

Old-fashioned gardeners discovered that when it was set near wilted dying plants in a garden, the drooping ones revived and grew green and healthy again.

Chamomile oil mixed with date sugar is an ancient Arabian and Egyptian remedy used to revive man's flagging energy and to relieve coughs and hoarseness. It is small enough to tote along on a camel trip through the desert, a barge journey down the Nile, or wherever your travels take you.

A dose of this convenient remedy, which I've carried on lecture tours—for quick energy and to prevent hoarseness—is a teaspoonful of date sugar moistened with six drops of chamomile oil.

Chamomile oil is not always available, so if you want to make your own, here's an old-fashioned recipe from *The Good House-Wife's Handbook of 1588:*

> *To make Oil of Chamomile:* Take one pint-and-a-half of cooking oil, and three ounces of chamomile flowers dried one day after they are gathered. Then put the oil and the flowers in a glass jar. Cover tightly. Let stand for forty days in the rays of the sun. (Old English of original text modernized.)

> *Modern variation:* Take safflower oil, a pint and a half, and three ounces of dried leaves from a package of chamomile tea. Put the oil and the tea in a glass or stainless steel saucepan, cover and simmer slowly for forty minutes. Remove from fire and let stand overnight. Strain and bottle.

In France, chamomile oil is used as a skin cleanser and tissue-strengthening lotion for the face, to massage swollen glands in the neck, to rub on painful joints, and to use warm as eardrops. A compress of chamomile tea is applied hot to aching joints, cold to bruises and sprains, and warm to eczema and other skin irritations.

In Ireland, chamomile tea is used to treat alcoholics suffering from delirium tremens. And for nerve exhaustion in both tipplers and nontipplers, the Irish favor a tea made of equal parts of chamomile and sage.

In Germany, chamomile tea is highly regarded as a soothing, relaxing drink and is used to treat headache, stomach distress, and minor kidney, bladder, spleen, and gallstone complaints.

An older generation of herbalists have reported instances of gallstones being dissolved by the continuous use of chamomile tea with lemon. And, more recently, modern German researchers have found that drinking chamomile tea can double the flow of bile. Here are some of the herb tea combinations used in Germany:

> *For Sick Headache and Nervous Stomach:* Equal parts of chamomile, mint, and catnip tea.
>
> *As a Mild Laxative and a Tonic for the Intestines and Minor Liver Complaints:* Equal parts of chamomile and comfrey tea with one teaspoonful of powdered bark of cascara sagrada dissolved in each cup.
>
> *For Minor Kidney Disorders and to Promote the Flow of Bile:* One part chamomile tea, two parts dandelion tea, and a generous squeeze of fresh lemon juice.

I have none of the ailments mentioned above, but I drink chamomile tea anyway. I like the taste of it, and I enjoy its unique relaxing effect when I've been working under pressure. Sometimes, when I'm drinking a cup of it, I think of a line from one of Edna St. Vincent Millay's poems, ". . . they always said tea was such a comfort." Indeed it is. Especially when it's comfrey or chamomile tea.

Fortunately for those of us who have neither the time nor the inclination to grow our own, comfrey and chamomile teas, ready for brewing, are available in health-food stores. And, as an added convenience, these teas are also prepared in premeasured tea bags ready to be dropped into a cup of hot water . . . so you can, with great ease, enjoy all the comforts of comfrey and chamomile.

COMFREY AND CHAMOMILE REMEDIES

**Coughs
and
Congestion**

Culpeper's Syrup of Comfrey

Take of comfrey root 6 ounces; plantain leaves, 3 ounces. Bruise together in a marble mortar to press out the juice; strain the liquid and add an equal quantity of honey. *Dose:* 2 tablespoonfuls.

Chlorophyll-Comfrey Tonic Soup—From France

To 1 cup of chopped comfrey leaves and 3 cups of one or more fresh salad greens that are in season, add 1 quart of buttermilk, 3 diced cucumbers, ½ cup chopped green onions, and 1 cup of yogurt. Blend until the mixture is smooth. Serve chilled, topped with a dollop of yogurt and a sprinkle of chives.

Herbal Nervine—From England

Simmer ⅓ cup of fresh, chopped celery (stalk *and* leaves) in 2½ cups of boiling water fifteen minutes. Strain. Put 1 heaping teaspoonful each of chamomile and hops tea in a preheated teapot. Reheat celery liquid to boiling, pour over the tea, cover and steep five minutes. *Dose:* ½ to 1 cupful twice a day, or as needed.

Chamomile-Lime Flower-Licorice Tonic— From Lebanon

In a preheated 2-cup teapot, put a small piece of licorice root and 1 teaspoonful each (or 1 tea bag each) of chamomile and lime flower tea. Fill teapot with freshly boiling water, cover, steep five minutes. May be drunk either hot or cold, as often as needed. When licorice root isn't available, either liquid or powdered licorice may be used.

Tonic for Female Debility—From Greece

3 tablespoons juniper berries
3 cups boiling water
1 teaspoon each of chamomile and comfrey tea (or 1 tea bag of each)
1 one-inch piece of licorice root

Wash the juniper berries and soak in cold water to cover for fifteen minutes. Drain and simmer for thirty minutes in 3 cups of boiling water, or until the water is reduced to 2 cups. Remove the berries. Place chamomile, comfrey, and licorice in a preheated teapot. Reheat the juniper berry liquid to boiling and pour over the tea. Cover and steep for five minutes. *Recommended dose:* Divide the 2 cups of liquid into 4 portions and take ½ cupful four times a day.

17

Medicine from the Sea Around Us

One of the most interesting aspects of folk remedies is their evolution. Some—like the rare seeds and herbs—are husbanded for one purpose only—medicine. Others—like honey or yogurt— are included in the national diet, their medicinal values remembered as little more than conversation pieces. For the most part, however, when a food's remedial properties are recognized— and it also happens to taste good—it becomes not only a meal-time staple but also a preventive confection, a snack—even a candy.

Never was this fact more apparent to me than when I visited Scotland, as a student, nearly half a century ago. When I arrived in Glasgow, one of the first sights that caught my eye was the large number of peddlers hawking some native delicacy that they wheeled along the streets in barrows. It went by a native name that I couldn't translate. Even the poorest people laid out pennies for this delicacy, served up in a rolled paper poke.

This "candy," I soon discovered, was nothing more than chopped seaweed! Still moist, it gave off a salty fragrance that added refreshment to its delightful taste. Traveling from one Scottish port city to another, I spent many a penny for this native snack—and have since wished fervently that it would catch on in the United States and other lands.

For I couldn't help thinking that the Scots' lifelong habit of eating seaweed—rich in silicon, sulfur, and other minerals—was largely responsible for the luxuriant hair and lovely complexion of their women. I also remembered that in ancient China, when long fingernails were a mark of the wealthy aristocrat, the Chinese drank a strong brew made of seaweed to strengthen their fingernails and make them grow faster.

Seaweed appears in more than four hundred different varieties. The most familiar variety is kelp, which grows abundantly along the coastlines of the North Atlantic and North Pacific oceans, the borders of lagoons and the inlets between islands, and along other coastlines in many parts of the world. Kelp also goes by the names of bladder wrack, bladder fucus, kelpware, sea wrack, sea oak, and our lady's wrack.

The last name, "our lady's wrack," came from an Irish legend about a girl who slipped and fell on a seawashed rock. She lay there, "wracked" with pain, her leg sprained so badly that she was unable to move away from the rising tide. Noticing the kelp that grew within her reach, she gathered a handful, bit open the tiny "bladders," and repeatedly rubbed her injured leg with their gelatinous substance. Relief from pain came rapidly enough for her to hobble to safety and wait for help to arrive.

Today in Ireland, the healing power of our lady's wrack is still credited with saving the girl's life. Irish fishermen still slit open the tiny bladders to rub on weak arm and leg muscles.

Throughout all the British Isles, kelp is regarded as a builder and strengthener of muscles. In Yorkshire fishing villages, mothers rub their infants' legs with a mixture of kelp and alcohol to prevent bowleggedness. In the coastal ports of England, Scotland, and Ireland, the same mixture is applied to ease the pains of lumbago or rheumatism, and to relieve the soreness of sprains, strained muscles, and ligaments.

Years after my first visit to Scotland, a group of naturalists and I were given permission to visit Ailsa Craig, a lighthouse island on the southwest coast, to study the many types of seaweed growing there. As we explored the inlets and borders of Ailsa Craig and examined the profusion of sea vegetation, it was easy to believe that during the Napoleonic Wars, when sodium was scarce, the quantity of mineral-rich kelp, gathered for commercial use in Scotland alone, amounted to 20,000 tons.

But the use of seaweed goes back many centuries before the days of Napoleon. Its merits as food and medicine were first recorded around 3000 B.C. by the Chinese emperor, Shen-nung.

During the time of Confucius, sea vegetation was so highly regarded that it was offered as sacrificial food for the gods.

Today we know that the calcium, sulfur, and silicon in kelp are important factors in keeping the fingernails strong and healthy. Silicon also increases the natural beauty of the skin and prolongs its youth by keeping the tissues firm and preventing sags and wrinkles. Cosmetic manufacturers have discovered the benefits of kelp and carrageen in beauty products. If you read the fine print listing the ingredients, you'll find that kelp and carrageen are used in many lotions, creams, and antiwrinkle preparations.

Kelp's iodine content is useful in restoring vigor and mental alertness, when their loss is caused by a sluggish thyroid. When the same loss results from iron-deficiency anemia, kelp's iron, copper, and zinc content help correct it. And a recent report by Dr. Joseph M. Kadans indicates that manganese and other minerals make kelp beneficial to the brain tissue, the sensory nerves, and the membrane surrounding the brain and spinal cords.

In China's neighboring country, Tibet, natives believe that "the strength of the gods" is in kelp. To gain the benefit of that strength, Tibetan guides carry small bags of dried kelp with them. When their muscles grow strained from hours of mountain climbing, or the high altitude causes shortness of breath or labored breathing, a pinch of kelp is their standard remedy to reduce the strain, ease the breathing difficulty, and renew their energy.

The ancients of Japan placed such a high value on seaweed, as both food and medicine, that they called it "heaven grass." In the thriving, industrial Japan of today, the harvesting of "heaven grass" and other sea vegetation has become a flourishing industry.

Diving girls, not men, are trained to explore the borders of coasts and offshore lagoons in search of seaweed. (The Japanese, proud of these superbly built, hardily conditioned divers, believe that women can hold their breaths longer than men and are better able to withstand the rigors of the ice-cold depths.)

With seaweed included in their everyday diet, the Japanese have little need for remedies containing it. In Japan, this plant is used in more diverse ways and the consumption of it is higher than in any other nation. Kelp, carrageen (Irish moss), and other forms of seaweed are used in soup, noodles, fish and vegetable dishes, baby foods, relishes, cookies, cakes, and puddings.

Significantly, in the Orient and other countries where the use of seaweed in the diet is above average, goiter and other abnormalities of the thyroid are almost unknown. The reason is that the iodine in kelp is a sure preventive against goiter.

Oriental women are noted for their slender figures, and the large amount of seaweed in their diet may be one of the factors contributing to their slimness. Kelp's value as a safe, mild diuretic eliminates the excess fluid stored in the tissues that results in water-weight, swelling, and a fat, bloated look. Its high iodine content has a normalizing effect on the thyroid, which can prevent or correct the weight-gain caused by a thyroid deficiency.

And kelp has a special antifat benefit for those who burn calories so slowly that they gain weight even when they eat very little. The body's metabolism controls the rate at which calories are burned. By stepping up a slow rate of metabolism, kelp speeds the burning of excess calories.

In European folk medicine, kelp, carrageen, and other types of seaweed have a long history of use as a digestive aid, an acidosis preventive, and a bowel cleanser. For these conditions, English coast dwellers brew a strong kelp decoction. Along the Irish shores, carrageen is preferred to kelp, and boiled milk is often substituted for water.

Seaweed is a storehouse of all the minerals considered vital to health, and many others whose functions in human nutrition are still under scrutiny. It contains mannitol, a gentle, natural laxative and bile stimulant, small amounts of lecithin, considered by many, including myself, as the greatest nutritional discovery in fifty years, vitamin A, some of the B-complex vitamins, and vitamins C and E.

The lecithin in kelp is known to be a fat emulsifier that aids in preventing and removing fatty deposits from the arteries. This is one reason why, in Japan and Scandinavia, kelp has been reported useful in cleansing the arteries, preventing the thickening and narrowing caused by fat blockage.

As medicine for the heart, seaweed had a long history among Indian tribes that inhabited coastal America. Each time a storm washed kelp onto the California shore, Costanoan medicine men sent their apprentices to gather it up. Dried and pulverized, it was fed to tribesmen complaining of chest pains or palpitations. In the territory that was later to become Rhode Island, Narragansett braves fought shortness of breath by chewing on fresh weed. The Tekestas and Calusas of Florida drank seaweed decoctions as general heart tonics.

Dulse, another variety of seaweed, was widely used by tribes of the Northeast. Penobscot shamans simmered it in seawater until it was reduced to a jellylike mass, then fed it to sufferers of heart ailments and rubbed it on their chests. Passamaquoddy warriors carried bags of dried, shredded dulse, which they nibbled on at the first signs of fatigue.

Descendants of Peruvian Indians, high in the Andes Mountains, still carry out a tradition of their forefathers. At regular intervals, they travel to the coast and bring back kelp; this journey lasts about a month. These people believe, simply, that kelp is "food for the heart."

Of course, professional diagnosis and advice should always be sought by those who already have a heart condition. But as a preventive measure, kelp may be taken safely by anyone. Rich in vitamins, minerals, and trace elements that benefit the heart, it can be of great value when combined with exercise and a proper diet.

The many folk uses of kelp have led to still another breakthrough in modern medicine. Each year in the United States, some 65,000 women develop breast cancer, and countless others live in fear of it. Now a Philadelphia scientist gives us reason to hope that this dreaded disease may be prevented by adding supplementary iodine to the daily diet.

In extensive tests on laboratory animals, and in preliminary clinical studies with humans, Dr. Bernard A. Eskin, of the Medical College of Pennsylvania, has compiled substantial evidence that iodine deficiency may contribute to the development of breast cancer and that sufficient amounts of iodine may aid in its prevention.

It's been known for some time that the incidence of breast cancer is higher in endemic goiter regions of the world, *i.e.*, areas where goiter is prevalent because the soil and food lack iodine. These locales, in which death rates from breast cancer are unusually high, include what's known in the United States as the "goiter belt"—the Great Lakes region and other parts of the Midwest—and the endemic goiter areas of Australia, Mexico, Poland, Russia, Switzerland, and Thailand.

"The similarity of high mortality regions to endemic goiter areas is striking," says Dr. Eskin. His statement is backed by evidence that neither goiter nor breast cancer are common in Iceland, where iodine-rich seafood constitutes a large part of the diet, or in Japan, which has a high consumption of both seafood and seaweed.

In his clinical studies of women with breast dysplasia (cysts, nodules, and abnormal tissue changes that can lead to cancer) Dr. Eskin reports that in every case where adequate iodine therapy was given, the condition decreased or disappeared.

"The treatment," he said, "seemed to be effective and at least temporarily improved the breast condition." While further research is necessary before conclusions can be drawn, Dr. Eskin has surely opened up the *possibility* of using iodine as a breast cancer preventive.

The United States Public Health Service has given grants to two research firms that will cultivate seaweed in germ-free environments and study the different varieties for their anticancer agents in general. Then, according to the National Cancer Institute, extracts from the varieties of seaweed will undergo comprehensive tests on cancers in animals.

Until the findings are complete, one could do a lot worse than to add this ancient folk remedy to his diet. Like all medicinal plants, seaweed is packed with nutrition, and it is loaded with more health-giving elements, perhaps, than any other food known to man.

KELP REMEDIES FROM
AROUND THE WORLD

**Muscle
Strengtheners**
Muscle Strengthener—From Yorkshire

3 cups kelp
rubbing alcohol

Wash kelp thoroughly to remove sea salt. Divide the bladders and cut into inch-long pieces. Place in a quart jar or bottle with a lid with enough alcohol to cover. Let stand, tightly covered, for a week. Shake well several times a day. Do not strain. Massage the lotion gently but firmly on weak muscles.

Skin Beautifiers

Seaweed Skin Beautifier—From Scotland

1 ounce carrageen
11 ounces distilled water
2 ounces glycerine
⅛ ounce boric acid
1 ounce eau de cologne

Wash carrageen in cold water. Place in a saucepan, add 10 ounces of distilled water, cover and simmer gently until carrageen is dissolved. Strain. Dissolve the glycerine and boric acid in the remaining ounce of water, cool and add cologne.

Stomach Aids

Kelp Digestive Aid—From England (and Ireland)

4 ounces kelp
2 quarts water

Wash kelp and chop into small pieces, leaving the bladders intact. Simmer slowly in water thirty minutes, or until liquid is reduced to one quart. Cool and strain.

Dose: One cupful every morning on arising, or half an hour before breakfast.

An Irish variation of the above substitutes carrageen (Irish moss) for kelp. For greater benefits, add ⅓ cup of boiled milk.

Lelord Kordel "Modern" Variation

1 ounce powdered kelp
1 quart boiling water

Place powdered kelp in a teapot, pour the boiling water over it and let steep, covered, for ten minutes.

Dose: One cup night and morning. More if needed.

**As a
Dessert**

Carrageen Orange Fruit Mold

> 1 ounce carrageen
> 1 quart water
>   juice of two lemons
> 1 pint fresh orange juice
>   honey
>   yogurt

Soak carrageen in cold water, drain, when softened, and place in a saucepan. Cover with boiling water. Simmer slowly thirty to forty minutes, or until seaweed is dissolved. Strain through a sieve, pressing through as much of the seaweed residue as possible. Add the lemon juice, orange juice, and honey, to taste. Pour into molds and refrigerate. When set, serve topped with a tablespoonful of yogurt. Add diced fresh fruit if you like.

18

Sex Stimulants and Hormone Boosters

Is impotence more prevalent in today's society than it was fifty years ago? The evidence indicates that it is, even among younger men. Or, if we can believe statistics, *especially* among younger men. Researchers tell us that in spite of the sexual "revolution," *performance* is at a surprisingly low ebb.

What's the reason for it?

In about 90 percent of the cases, decreased sexual ability is psychologically caused. But, as a nutritionist, I have witnessed another common reason: poor eating habits. At any age, an undernourished body doesn't give its hormones a fighting (and loving!) chance.

A slowdown of hormone production can throw the glandular system out of balance. Dr. William H. Masters, gynecologist, pioneer in sexual physiology, and author of *Human Sexual Response,* confirms my teachings when he says that when an individual stays in negative protein balance his sex drive diminishes. Impotence "often reflects a hormone deficiency," he stated.

Some of the foods the ancients prescribed as aphrodisiacs are based on that premise. Glandular meats, fish, eggs, and honey were high on their list, and so were many herbs, seeds, nuts, fruits, and vegetables.

Garlic and onion were considered powerful sexual stimulants, and Ovid included "the white shallots sent from Megara" in a compilation of aphrodisiacs. Another early Roman poet, Martial, gave this endorsement of onions:

"If envious age relax the nuptial knot
Thy food be scallions and thy feast shallot."

A Moslem recipe for sexual prowess combined onions, eggs, and spices. First the onions were simmered in water with spices, then browned in oil and served with egg yolk.

Sheikh Nefzawi, in *The Perfumed Garden,* favored creamed chicken broth with egg yolks and powdered almonds to restore virility. Other Arabian invigorators consisted of egg yolks, saffron and asparagus, and a mixture of milk and honey.

Hormone precursors help improve the function of your glands by boosting hormone production. Judicious use of true hormone-containing plants, combined with a diet that includes hormone precursors, should provide enough hormones to maintain virility and prevent impotency under normal conditions.

For more than thirty years, scientists have been searching for hormones and hormone precursors in plants. Two American researchers, Professor Russell E. Marker and Dr. Aval Rohrman, of Pennsylvania State College, tested hundreds of plants in their search for natural sources, but each analysis ended in disappointment.

It was in Mexico, in 1939, that they began to experiment with extracts from sarsaparilla roots. After careful analysis, they announced their discovery: *Sarsaparilla root contains hormones!*

To students of folk medicine, this came as no great surprise. It has long been known that in the Orient, and in tropical areas of Central and South America, sarsaparilla's native habitats, the roots are made into a pleasant-tasting tea for sexual virility. And American Indians considered sarsaparilla root one of their most valuable sex remedies.

In Paris some years ago, I noticed that many women, in hotels and restaurants, drank the same beverage. It was a clear liquid that looked and smelled like anisette. My waiter at a sidewalk café told me that it was licorice water. Knowing that licorice is considered a blood purifier that benefits the skin, I asked, "Do they drink it to improve their complexions?"

"No, no, Monsieur," he said. "To improve their love life!"

Did the Frenchwomen know something about licorice that scientists were not to discover until several years later? Perhaps . . . for soon afterward came the news that female hormones had been found in licorice!

You can make your own "French licorice water" by mixing a spoonful of powdered licorice (available in health-food stores) in a glass of plain soda. Commercially prepared licorice confections are available in some form in most stores, but try to choose those with the least amount of sugar.

The ancient East has been years ahead of Europeans in knowing how to maintain and restore male potency. From the *Kama Sutra* comes this priceless information:

1. "A man obtains sexual vigour by drinking milk mixed with honey, the root of the uchchata plant, the pipar chaba, and liquorice."
2. Mix together: ghee [clarified butter], honey, liquorice, the juice of the fennel plant, and milk in equal quantities. This nectar-like composition is said to be provocative of sexual vigor."

Pollen has been known as a unique source of energy for centuries. Both Pliny and Virgil had confidence in its ability to invigorate the male, aid in maintaining his virility, and protect him from some of the diseases associated with aging.

The success of pollen in treating prostate trouble has become a matter of record. More recently, Dr. Alois Schusta, a gynecologist of Vienna, reported remarkable results among women patients with female disorders.

The women, ranging in age from twenty-nine to fifty-nine, suffered from nervous disorders, insomnia, menopause or premenopause complaints, and physical and sexual debility. All of the patients had failed to respond to previous treatment, but after two eight-day courses of treatment with pollen tablets, 90 percent were cured. Those who required a longer course of treatment were greatly improved. In both groups, the lasting effects of the cure, unlike that of some therapy, continued after treatment had stopped.

What unknown biochemical makes pollen beneficial in prostate and other male disorders, the ailments commonly called "female trouble," and physical and sexual weakness in both sexes? What else except a combination of male and female hormones?

Three members of the faculties of biochemistry and pharmacy at the University of Zagreb recently reported that they had found the male hormone, testosterone, in pollen, along with traces of epitestosterone and androstenedione. The quantities they discovered were minute, but enough to give a needed boost to the body's own production of hormones when it begins to slow down—a safe, natural boost, with long-lasting results and no harmful side effects.

In England, hops tea and tonic water are still widely used to relieve headache and stomach distress, induce sleep, as a general tonic to strengthen the body, and as a nervine. (Tonic water is also known as quinine water.)

British researchers, investigating the merits of folk remedies, have found that hops lives up to most of the ancient claims made for it and the faith that an increasing number of modern women have in it. In addition to its other virtues, it acts as a stimulant to the muscles and glands, including the sex glands, which receive a gentle boost from hops' natural estrogen content. Though it's only a minute amount, it's enough to give noticeable results when added to the body's own hormone production, especially when that production begins to slow down.

British women drink hops tea neat ("straight"), but the majority of men seem to prefer it mixed with an English tea. And the entire family is given a homemade hops tonic as a general conditioner, hormone booster, and nerve tonic anytime it's needed.

Generations of Gypsies have favored hops remedies for a wide variety of women's ailments, and as a nervine, invigorator, and general tonic for all of the men, women, and children of their tribes.

Nursing mothers drink hops tea to increase breast milk and for its soothing effect on the nervous system. Older women drink the tea and a tonic made of hops and other herbs to help them through the discomforts of the menopause. The elderly depend upon both the tea and the tonic as a "strengthener" that gives them a feeling of well-being, and Gypsy men of all ages believe that both beverages promote male and female sexual vigor.

At this time, sarsaparilla, licorice, pollen, and hops are the only known natural sources of male and/or female hormones in measurable amounts. Many others have been used for centuries, as aphrodisiacs, but science has yet to uncover actual hormones in them.

For thousands of years, the Chinese and other Asians have regarded ginseng as their most potent health restorer and general rejuvenator, not only of the sex glands but of the entire body. In China, the old and sick drink a daily cup of ginseng tea or a decoction made of the roots, to restore their health and vigor, and the young and healthy drink it to retain these attributes.

The ancient medical book of India, *The Atherva Veda,* says that ginseng is an aid in producing "seed that is poured into the female that forsooth is the way to bring forth a son." And another hope it holds out is that ". . . this herb will make thee so full of lusty strength that thou shalt, when thou art excited, exhale heat as a thing on fire."

Modern herbalists have reported the successful use of ginseng in treating patients suffering from a general rundown condition; mental, physical, and emotional exhaustion (all of which can cause temporary impotency) ; and sexual debility. It may not make you "exhale as a thing on fire," but tests have shown that ginseng contains tonic properties, exerts a beneficial influence on the central nervous system, and does indeed have a stimulating effect on both the male and female sex glands.

From the jungles of the Eastern Tropics comes another plant regarded as a "wonder herb" by Asians: *hydrocotyle Asiatica.* The legend of its invigorating and rejuvenating powers dates back to antiquity, and within recent years both the French and British governments decided to test its accuracy.

The plant was found to contain unique tonic and revitalizing properties. These substances, like those in ginseng, have a stimulating effect on the endocrine gland system and act as a natural aid in restoring and maintaining the healthful functioning of the sex glands.

Doctors in India and China generally prescribe a tea or decoction made of the leaves, but the majority of the people use the entire plant—twigs, leaves, root, and seeds. In India, a remedy for general and sexual weakness is made by simmering equal parts of Hydrocotyle Asiatica and licorice root in milk.

Asafetida also has a long, impressive record in folk medicine. We know it mostly as an odorous gumlike substance that used to be worn in a bag around the neck to ward off colds, but Asians value it for its tonic properties and as a stimulant and aphrodisiac.

In Asia, the thick, reddish gum-resin that exudes when the

plant is cut is scraped off into a container, allowed to harden in the sun, and is then reduced to a powder. An ounce of the powder, stirred into a pint of boiling water, makes a tonic that is taken a tablespoonful at a time to produce the desired results.

An analysis of asafetida has shown that among its many beneficial factors are those that tend to stimulate the brain, nervous system, and glands, as most well-known sex gland stimulants do.

Gobernadora is another plant that contains valuable resins. Indians and Mexicans of the Coahuila Province chew the leaves or make them into a tea to be used as an aphrodisiac.

In Turkey and Syria, two types of orchids, *Orchis mascula* and *Orchis latifolia,* are cultivated for their nutritive, nervine, tonic, and hormone-boosting properties. The fresh roots are washed and dipped into hot water, and the outer skin is rubbed off with a cloth. The blanched roots are then spread on a tin plate or cookie sheet and baked from eight to ten minutes, or until they lose their opaque quality and acquire a slightly transparent look.

British herbalist Mrs. C. F. Leyel tells this legend about them: "The name satyrion, which is used for the orchid, is derived from the belief that the flower was the food of the satyrs, and induced the sexual excesses to which they were prone."

Dates—a sexual stimulant? We know them as a delicious fruit, high in food and energy value, but in Arabia, Egypt, and Iran, dates are highly regarded both as an important source of sustenance and as a sexual invigorator.

Asians make a distillation of tree-ripened dates called *lagbi,* or *rajura-no-darn,* which has a decided sex-stimulating action. Also in Asia, a single date palm tree produces an abundance of sap, which, when left to ferment, forms another spirit called arrack, that has the same effect as *lagbi.*

The Pawnee Indians, like generations of Orientals, favored a decoction of ginseng root as a tonic, stimulant, and invigorator, especially for Indian males. A combination used by both men and women of the tribe, but considered especially beneficial to the male, was made by simmering ginseng root with wild columbine and parsley. Men of the Omaha and Ponca tribes used a decoction of wild columbine seeds as a tonic to increase sexual desire and vigor.

Two flower remedies were highly regarded as sexual stimulants by the Navajo Indians of the Southwest. A strong tea, made of the ephemeral blossoms of the day-flower, was drunk to increase the desire of the women and the potency of the men. The same tribe used an infusion of lupine blossoms as a sexual stimulant and remedy for sterility.

Damiana is widely known as a treatment for sexual weakness and impotency and is reported to strengthen the organs of reproduction. It's also used as a tonic for the nervous system, and is said to have good results in treating physical, mental, and nervous exhaustion.

In California, Mexico, the West Indies, and South America, damiana leaves are gathered, dried, and shipped to the rest of the world. The recommended method of preparation is to pour a cup of boiling water over a teaspoonful of the dried leaves (or one-fourth teaspoonful of ground leaf powder). *Dose:* A tablespoonful two or three times a day.

If you live along the southern California coast or the southeastern shores from Georgia to Florida, you can pick your own fresh saw palmetto berries from this short, stemless palm that has won worldwide fame in folk medicine.

Widely known as a tonic to the mucous membranes, the tissues and glands, including the sex glands, it has a direct influence on the organs of reproduction. Four or five fresh berries, eaten three times a day, are recommended for normalizing and stimulating underactive sex glands and improving their function.

In women, regular use of the berries is said to normalize the mammary glands, resulting in firmness and either an increase or decrease in the size of breasts that have grown flabby and are either too small or too large.

If dried berries or powder are used, the recommended infusion, for both men and women, is made by pouring one-half pint of boiling water over an ounce of the dried herb. Let steep until cool, bottle, and take one teaspoonful three times a day.

From ancient Greeks, Romans, and Chinese to modern Russians, Asians, and members of other countries around the world, sunflower seeds have been eaten as a source of male vigor and potency.

Pumpkin seeds, favored by male Gypsies as a hormone booster for many generations, are now known to be of special benefit in restoring and maintaining the healthful functioning of the prostate gland.

Sunflower seeds and pumpkin seeds, hulled for easy eating, can be carried in the pocket for between-meal energizers, as Roman soldiers used to do on their long marches, while dreaming of beautiful conquests!

In ancient Babylon, women ate confections made of sesame seeds and honey to increase their sexual desire and fertility. (They fed them to the men, too!) Modern French and American researchers have found that a sesame seed-honey combination has excellent results in boosting lowered vitality and sexual energy.

Lady's mantle has long been known as "a woman's best friend." A tea made of the dried herb is an old-time remedy for various women's ailments. Once highly regarded as a protector and revitalizer for female organs, it is said to be of special value in improving their functions during the menopause and afterward, when female hormone production decreases.

The feathery-leaved fennel, with a scent reminiscent of new-mown hay, was known as the "Pearl of Aphrodisiacs" by the ancients.

The leaves are the part most widely used today, but in Algeria I have eaten the pale hearts of fennel shoots cooked as a vegetable that reminded me of artichoke hearts. (And artichoke hearts remind me of their merits described by Paris street vendors who used to cry, "Artichokes! Artichokes! Heats the body and the spirit. Heats the genitals!")

In England, where fennel is grown in many home gardens, both the fresh and dried leaves are used for tea. For a stronger decoction, the bruised or finely crushed seeds are simmered in water and drunk as a tea or used as a remedy in combination with other ingredients. Crushed fennel seeds, combined with licorice root, are part of a popular British commercial preparation affectionately known as "tonic for happy lovers." (See recipes at the end of chapter.)

France's famous plant-healer, Maurice Messegue, recommends a variety of herbs, in personally supervised amounts, for both male and female sexual debility. Among them are many of those already mentioned and others that are widely used in this country, including the crushed seeds of fenugreek and the leaves of greater celandine, peppermint, summer savory, and sage, for both men and women, prepared as a tea, a decoction, a tincture, or a tonic.

In addition, he recommends broad-leaved plantain for women and buttercup leaves and blossoms for men.

From the ancients to the moderns, meat has been unanimously endorsed to restore and retain virility. In researcher Jeanne Rose's herbal compendiums, two words stand out in a list of known sexual stimulators: *meat diet.*

Havelock Ellis, a famous British scientist and sexologist, considered beefsteak "as powerful a sexual stimulant as any food."

And in the *Satyricon,* Encolpius tells of his virility booster before keeping a date with Circe, the enchantress: "To encourage my jaded body . . . I apply'd myself to strong meats . . . strong broth and eggs, using wine moderately . . ." It was good advice in ancient times, just as it is today.

Oriental Virility Cocktail

2 ounces sarsaparilla root
powdered or ground ginger
1 quart water

Bring the root and water to boil, cover and simmer slowly for one half hour. Cool and strain. When ready to serve, add a fleck of ginger to each glass. May be drunk hot or cold.

Dose: One wineglassful three or four times a day, or as often as needed.

Compound for Increasing Energy and Sexual Vigor— From Arabia

3 tablespoons sesame seed
1 ounce licorice root
1/4 pound dates, pitted and finely chopped
2 quarts water
1 cup honey

Simmer first three ingredients in water until the liquid is reduced to 1 quart. Remove from fire and add honey, stirring until mixture is thoroughly blended.

Dose: 2 tablespoonfuls three or four times a day, or as needed for an energizer and hormone booster.

Hops Family Tonic—From England

3 tablespoons dried hops
   (or hops tea)
Peel of 2 lemons, washed and
   sliced

Peel of 1 orange, washed and
   sliced
1 quart water
Honey to taste
3 tablespoons lecithin granules

Simmer lemon and orange peel in water twenty minutes. Add hops and simmer three minutes. Remove from fire and stir in honey. Cover and allow to cool to lukewarm. Strain. Add lecithin and mix well.

Dose: Wineglassful, three or four times a day.

Gypsy Herbal Invigorator

1 ounce hops
1 ounce alfalfa
1 ounce agrimony
1 ounce centaury
1 quart water

Mix the herbs well, add water, bring to a boil. Cover and simmer fifteen minutes. Remove from fire, cool and strain. Sweeten with honey, if desired.

Dose: One-half cupful before meals, three times daily. (All of the herbs are available in health-food stores.)

American Indian Love Tonic

2 tablespoons unrefined oatmeal
½ cup raisins
1 quart water
Honey
Juice of 2 lemons

Bring first three ingredients to a boil. Reduce heat, cover tightly, and simmer slowly forty-five minutes. Remove from fire and strain. To the resulting liquid, stir in honey to taste. (Save the oatmeal and raisins for the children's breakfast.) When cool, add lemon juice. Refrigerate to use as needed.

Dose: At least two cups a day, preferably one before breakfast and another at bedtime. If you're an insomniac, it helps that unhappy condition as well!

Babylonian Revitalizer for Both Sexes
(Kordel version with wheat germ and powdered milk)

1 cup sesame seeds
¾ cup honey
½ cup wheat germ
Powdered skim milk

Mix sesame seeds, honey, and wheat germ thoroughly. Add powdered milk a spoonful at a time, kneading it well into other ingredients until mixture has the consistency of firm dough. (Amount of powdered skim milk used depends upon whether honey is thick or thin. Thin honey requires additional solid substances to make it "hold together.") Shape into walnut-sized balls, roll in more powdered skim milk or wheat germ to prevent stickiness, and refrigerate until ready to eat. If you have a small grain mill or an old-fashioned coffee grinder, try grinding the sesame seeds into a meal and substitute that for the whole seeds to make a firmer-textured confection.

Tonic for Happy Lovers

2 teaspoons bruised fennel seeds
1 ounce licorice root
1 pint water

Combine all ingredients and bring to boil. Lower heat, cover, simmer slowly twenty minutes. Let stand until cool. Strain.
Dose: one to three tablespoonfuls twice a day.

19

Russian Secrets of Health and Super Energy

Conserving the famed energy of the Russian people, and keeping them fit, has been of great concern to Alexei A. Pokrovsky, director of the Soviet Academy's Institutes of Nourishment and Medical Sciences.

"We Russians tend to eat too much of everything, and we have some very overweight ladies and gentlemen to prove it" has been the essence of his message to the Soviet citizenry. "Very few of us work as hard as our forefathers, but we still eat as if we did! Strength and energy come from the *quality* of food we eat, not the *quantity!*"

"Don't be a starch casualty!" was another of his clarion calls that rattled the cake racks, shivered the bread bins, and warned the "overweight ladies and gentlemen" that gross changes—or changes from the gross—were part of his health and super-energy plan.

If the health hazards of a diet high in fats and carbohydrates were to be avoided, and if Russian energies were to be lifted and sustained at their characteristically high levels, the too, too solid flesh would have to be melted. This was the general opinion among Russia's doctors and nutritionists, but it was Alexei Pokrovsky who was doing something about it.

He proposed a new dietary balance high in protein, low in fats and carbohydrates, and *not to exceed a daily intake of 2,000 calories.* Any amount beyond 2,000 calories would be extended to only two groups: hard-training athletes and those whose work involved "very heavy manual labor." But even to those energy-burning members of the populace, margins of generosity would be narrow and grudging.

The Russian diet has always leaned to the more natural, unrefined foods, including an abundance of sauerkraut, pickled beets, buttermilk, yogurt, kefir, and other native sour-milk products. These lactic-acid foods are endorsed by Pokrovsky for their cleansing, health-promoting effect on the digestive tract as well as their energizing and revitalizing properties.

Russians are noted for their endurance, vitality, and longevity. The largest and best-documented group of centenarians lives in the Caucasus Mountains. Documented stories of men and women from the region show that they are healthy and vigorous, not only at one hundred, but some are still active at the validated age of one hundred and fifty and more.

The life-prolonging effect of mountain living was explained by the director of the Soviet Respiratory Laboratory. His theory is that aging is an effect of gradual asphyxiation caused by the progressive deterioration of the lungs. "In the mountains," he said, "air is rarefied, and keeps the lungs working with greater efficiency. Life tends to be automatically prolonged."

On my visit to the mountains I thought of this as I watched the Russian folk dancing and listened to their lively conversations and rich laughter. The group I was watching had already laid claim to the title of octogenarian. Now these folk were looking forward with active minds and bodies, clear vision and undisguised pleasure, to the hundredth candle on the birthday cake and the accolade of centenarian.

An old Russian proverb says, "For every disease there is a plant."

Today's Soviet scientists have won universal acclaim for their contributions to science; my observations confirmed the fact that herbal and natural remedies, not drugs, constitute 40 percent of the curative therapy of the Soviet Union. Among the long-lived mountain folk, where doctors are scarce, the figure would come closer to 100 percent.

Since ancient times, more than 1,000 plants, along with a few simple kitchen remedies, have been used for curative purposes in Russia. Some of these Russian folk remedies are given at the end of this chapter.

But back to Moscow, where, instead of scolding the Russian people, we find Alexei Pokrovsky in the kitchen! The scientist often dons the cook's apron when he experiments in his efforts to improve the Institute's "master food"—a low-cost, low-carbohydrate, energy-building fare of multi-benefits called Belip (an abbreviation of the Russian term for "Protein Development of the Nutrition Institute").

The basic ingredients of this super-energy food are inexpensive, and that alone is enough to recommend it in these days of soaring meat prices and the prospect of future shortages of protein foods.

Besides being high in proteins and minerals, Belip has other virtues which have earned it an important place on the menus of hospitals, school cafeterias, and restaurants noted for *healthful gourmet dishes.*

Belip is a must at athletes' training tables. In heavy industry, the workers' "break" is, more often than not, a break for Belip. Dancers replenish their spent energies with it. And among Russia's cosmonauts, Belip has become as important as their missions. Perhaps Belip can launch you from your pad. Or if you are grounded because you are beginning to get too pudgy, it could help you get rid of some of your *padding.*

Belip

1 pound codfish, skinned and boned	1 stalk celery, minced
1 pound cottage cheese (room temperature)	1 teaspoon dried dill weed
½ cup sunflower oil (or safflower oil)	1½ teaspoon sea salt (plain or seasoned)
1 large onion, minced	Freshly ground pepper to taste

Simmer the codfish in lightly salted water until flakes separate easily with fork. Drain, cool, then mash thoroughly, and add to the cottage cheese in a medium-large bowl. Sauté onion and celery in heated oil until crisply tender. Allow these to cool a bit, then combine, oil and all, with fish and cheese. Sprinkle mixture with dill weed, sea salt and pepper to taste, then blend *very thoroughly.* This energizing Russian health food is now ready to be served. Or try it in one of the following variations.

Belip Burgers: Shape into patties, allowing 4 ounces for each serving. Roll in toasted wheat germ and sautée in safflower oil until crisp and golden. May be served with tomato sauce.

Belip Balls: Allowing a generous tablespoon for each ball, roll between oiled hands, then dip in fresh, snipped parsley and chill thoroughly. Mayonnaise laced with sharp mustard makes an ideal accompaniment for these.

Belip Dumplings: Mix half of the recipe with one beaten egg. Form little dumplings and drop into hot chicken broth. Garnish with watercress and chopped green onions.

Longevity and active oldsters of the Caucasus Mountains were again brought into focus when the "roving researchist," Dr. Anna Kamerinskaya, and I strolled past a beautiful buckthorn tree growing on the clinic grounds.

"We call it 'Siberian Pineapple,'" she said. "When winter comes and the brilliant orange berries appear, my special pets at the clinic, the lively 'young' oldsters, will be out to harvest them. The oil from the berries is very healing. It makes a soothing application for external burns and sores. And I don't know of any berry that contains more vitamins C and P."

She continued, "A light tea made from one teaspoon of the bark is an enjoyable tonic, while a stronger tea, made from two teaspoons, acts as a gentle laxative."

When I teased the doctor gently about sounding like a folk practitioner, her answer was, "My dear colleague, to be really Russian is to have a remedy or more up your sleeve, down your boot, or under your pillow. In my case, it sometimes means sucking one up through a pipette, or shaking one around in a test tube."

I liked her approach in these matters, which, incidentally, seemed to be a general one among Soviet physicians. "We never close our eyes or our minds to folk remedies," she told me. "Recognizing that they formed the basis for modern medicine, we always test them."

Here are some of those Russian folk remedies which have been tested by time and usage:

Elixir of the Ukraine is a familiar and everyday booster of the energies of the vigorous older folk who live in and around Kharkov and Kiev. Many of them, still stepping out in sprightly fashion, can recall having taken this remedy first in their youth.

"The days of our labor were long and hard," one ninety-year-young man once told Dr. Kamerinskaya, "and we needed something to tone us up so we could bring the day to a happy close, with a little dancing and fun. I still take the elixir, doctor. I still dance, and I still have fun!"

You can make this Ukrainian lifter-upper very easily: Combine one pound of garlic, peeled and pulped, with the strained juice of two dozen fresh lemons. Heat thoroughly in an enameled pan, then add one pound of honey. Heat again just to the boiling point. Put the mixture in jars, cover loosely, set aside to cool. When cool, screw the lids fairly tightly and store your "elixir" in a warmish place for a ripening period of three weeks.

A tablespoonful of the mixture—be sure to shake it well—in a small glass of warm water is taken each evening during dinner. That is the *usual* way to take this invigorator, but I have learned to like it, without water, poured over salad greens or tomatoes.

Schizandra chinesis is the botanical name for the little roseate berries Russians call by the simpler name of limonik. Legend has it that hunters and trappers who had to put up for a time in the taiga, the swampy forest regions of Siberia, subsisted quite healthfully on nothing but these berries.

Happily for us, supplies are nearer than the swamps of Siberia. Chinese herbalists stock them routinely. A tea made from the dried berries could be the answer to your middle-of-the-afternoon droops. The berries make quite pleasant chewing.

Plantain leaves can be a soothing aid to throats that are sore from coughing or the too-lengthy discussion to which doctors, teachers, and lecturer-nutritionists are subject all too often. An infusion made of one tablespoonful of the leaves to one measuring cup of boiling water will yield enough to carry you over a period of two or three days. *Dose:* One tablespoon to be swallowed four times daily, preferably after meals.

Saint-John's-wort is recommended as being helpful in mild cases of colitis. One teaspoon of the dried herb added to eight ounces of boiling water will produce an efficacious infusion that is best taken after meals. Strain the mixture through cloth, not metal.

Ginseng could, quite feasibly, prove to be the most effective inhibitor of the aging process that we have encountered to date. "That would seem to be the essence of the reports that have come to my attention concerning the 'root of life,' as ginseng is known in the Soviet Union," said Dr. Kamerinskaya when I broached the topic of this remarkable herb.

"Admittedly, we do not speak from the vantage point of the centuries-old tradition of its use that the Chinese can boast, but we have been testing for its possible good effects over a period of some twenty years. As a result of our own research, I think we have some interesting things to say about it."

For example, there is a growing interest in its possibilities as a treatment for blood-pressure difficulties. The interest in this connection derives from the observation that it seems to exercise a beneficial influence on the central nervous system. As a gonadotrophic agent, it would also appear to have some merit, acting as a stimulus upon the sex glands without any harmful effects.

Ginseng's reputation as a useful tonic is reaching a point of scientific acclaim. Soviet pharmacologist, Dr. Ivan Brekham, has expressed the belief that the day is close when ginseng will be prescribed "as a matter of routine" for people of all ages who are not quite up to par.

Russia has a rich tradition of folk medicine, and someday I hope to have time for extended visits to other parts of this vast and interesting country.

As I said good-bye to my new Russian friends, Dr. Kamerinskaya asked me to have a final glass of Elixir of the Ukraine with them.

"You'll need it to prevent jet lag," she said, and raised her glass in a toast. "To you and the very good health of your people and mine . . . to *détente* . . . and an increasing exchange of ideas between our two countries!"

RUSSIAN REMEDIES FOR SPECIFIC PROBLEMS

For Arthritic, Rheumatic and Stiff Joint Pains

1. Place two pounds of fresh birch leaves (or one pound of dried) in a cotton bag or old pillowcase. Boil gently in two gallons of water forty minutes. Add both the bag and the birch water to a bathtub of comfortably hot water and soak for at least twenty minutes, adding more hot water as needed. (When birch leaves are not available, the same amount of pine needles make a relaxing, pain-easing substitute.)

2. Most of us know the efficacy of Epsom salts baths to relieve pain. But, according to reports, Russian results have proved more rapid and spectacular. The reason for this became clear when I learned that, when Russians soak in a tub of Epsom salts they don't fool around with a scant cup or two as we do. Five pounds are dissolved in a tub of hot water high enough to reach the armpits. (In old Russia deep oaken vats were used, and still are in some mountain regions.)

Liniment for Joint and Muscular Pains and Chest Congestion

⅓ teaspoon dry camphor
⅓ teaspoon dry mustard
1 pint turpentine
1 pint sunflower oil
1 pint rubbing alcohol

Dissolve camphor and mustard in the turpentine. Add sunflower oil (or other vegetable oil) and alcohol. Shake well before using. For best results, massage the painful area with liniment, allowing the skin to absorb all it can. Then apply a flannel or woolen wrapping.

Celery, Vinegar, and Kelp Tonic

For nerves, nervous headache, digestive disorders (especially when owing to a lack of hydrochloric acid), and as a general tonic.

1 pound celery, finely chopped
2 pints cider vinegar
1 tablespoon kelp granules

Place celery in a jar with a tightly fitting lid. Bring vinegar to a boil and remove at once from flame. Stir kelp granules in the hot vinegar and pour over the celery. Cover tightly. Keep closely stoppered.

Dose: Two teaspoonfuls in a half glass of hot or cold water, two or three times a day, preferably before meals.

Horseradish-Mustard Seed Decoction

This simple remedy is an excellent digestive aid and is recommended highly by old-timers for the relief of dropsy.

> 2 ounces horseradish root, scraped
> ½ ounce mustard seed, well bruised
> 1½ pints boiling water

Place horseradish and mustard seed in a jar. Pour boiling water over them. Cover. Let stand two hours. Strain.

Dose: Two tablespoonfuls, three times a day.

Liver Tonics

1. Beet juice, either by itself or mixed with a few drops of horseradish juice or the finely scraped root, is an old Russian folk remedy to "cleanse" and condition the liver. It's also said to have an equally beneficial effect on the kidneys.

Dose: One cup, two or three times a day.

2. Corn-silk tea, made of the silky strands under the leaves of fresh corn, is valued as a liver tonic and as a supplementary treatment for rheumatic patients. Boil one heaping teaspoonful of chopped corn silk in one and a half cups of water for ten minutes. Strain and drink hot, as often as needed, a cup at a time. May be sweetened with honey and flavored with a squeeze of lemon.

Pumpkin Seed Prostate Tonic

For inflammation of the bladder and prostate as well as other prostate disorders, simmer four ounces of *whole* (not shelled) pumpkin seeds in a quart of water twenty minutes. Cool and pour into a wide-mouthed bottle or jar. Do not strain. The seeds will settle to the bottom and may be discarded later.

Dose: A wineglassful, three times a day or whenever pain occurs. Be sure to stir thoroughly before using.

High Blood Pressure

In southern Russia and the Caucasus, garlic is used for high blood pressure, as it is in all of Russia. But in these regions, the lowly potato is highly regarded as a simple remedy.

Potato Peel Decoction. Simmer the well-washed peeling of five medium potatoes in a pint of water for twenty minutes. Cool and strain.

Dose: One cupful twice a day.

Hawthorn Berry Heart Tonic

Hawthorn berries have a long history of success in preventing arteriosclerosis and in benefitting such conditions as rapid and feeble heart action, heart valve defects, hypertrophy (enlargement) of the heart, angina pectoris, and difficult breathing owing to ineffective heart action and lack of oxygen in the blood.

In the Caucasus Mountains, Russian heart patients use the hawthorn berry in the following manner, preparing a fresh supply every day:

Pour two cups of boiling water over three tablespoonfuls of hawthorn berries. Cover and let stand overnight until midday in a very warm place (over a pilot light is fine). Strain the infusion through a fine mesh sieve or cloth, squeezing all juice from the berries.

Dose: One cup, taken with meals at least twice a day. For a three-cup-a-day treatment, increase the formula accordingly.

When fresh hawthorn berries are not available the dried or powdered fruit can be obtained in many herb and health-food shops.

20

Fifty Centuries of Chinese Folk Medicine

An old Chinese proverb states that "all men's diseases enter by way of his mouth." If that is so, then surely curatives and remedies must enter by the same opening.

This must have been Emperor Shen Nung's thinking when he wrote his *Pen Ts'ao,* the first book on natural and folk remedies. Many editions of his work were printed; this speaks well for the efficacy of the emperor's remedies.

But what speaks best for them is that the emperor, who tested his remedies on himself before recommending them to others, is reported to have lived one hundred and twenty-three healthy and productive years.

The recorded lore of Chinese folk medicine has expanded enormously since Shen Nung made the contribution that formed its basis. China has always had a more liberal attitude toward natural remedies than is true of Western thinking, and more particularly of officialdom's thinking. China's sixteenth-century pharmacopoeia, or Book of Remedies, is still in use. What augurs well for its contents is that Western men of the healing arts are looking ever more favorably to Chinese methods (both folk and orthodox) which have stood the test of recorded time— more than fifty centuries of it!

Through the years it has been my privilege to meet many Chinese practitioners of the healing arts. But my fondest memories are those of Dr. Lin Su Chan, whom I first met during my student days.

When I arrived for my first visit with Dr. Lin, he was busily tilling the garden in back of his house. This in itself wasn't strange, but the plants that grew there certainly were. Yet what else was I expecting? Why else had I come?

Dr. Lin was something of a legend. Possessing a long string of degrees in medicine and the sciences, he was as conversant with modern drug theory as with *yin* and *yang*. Frequently, surgeons and specialists consulted him, not only for his knowledge of ancient Oriental healing arts but also for his superb skills as an orthodox physician.

This odd combination of the ancient and the modern was what fascinated me most about Dr. Lin. The two just didn't seem to belong together. That first day we spent in his garden, I was more interested in the teacher than what he was about to teach. But what I learned about the *man* was really my first lesson in the subject. I queried him about the seeming conflict between folk healing and modern medicine.

Dr. Lin laughed as he said, "The conflict between folk healing and modern medicine? Why do you assume there must be a conflict?"

The first principle of Chinese medicine, he went on, is to learn and to share—to blend all knowledge. "For example," he said, pointing at a beautiful growth of heart-shaped leaves and purple flowers, "that plant has been in use for seven thousand years. Its Chinese name is *niu p'ang tze*—in America, it's known as the great burdock."

Dr. Lin then launched into a chemical analysis of the plant. All its parts, I learned, contain vitamin C, iron, and niacin. Fixed and volatile oils are also present in them, as are small amounts of mucilage, resin, and tannin.

"But you didn't come for a chemical analysis, I'm sure. I merely wish to point out why this plant is so well ensconced in the annals of Chinese folk medicine—as a blood purifier, a preventive of rheumatism, and as a benefit to those suffering from such chronic skin diseases as psoriasis and eczema. Its leaves and roots contain effective laxative and diuretic properties, while the seeds are rich in ingredients that prevent boils and styes. And that, my friend, is the last lesson you will ever receive from me about a single plant!"

I would have to find out for myself, he explained, and I soon understood why. Oriental folk medicine dates to primordial times—perhaps 20,000 years ago. At first, tribal healers experimented with simple cures, using the same trial-and-error methods as all ancient peoples. But, by about 3000 B.C., the folk methods began evolving into an organized system. And therein lies the difference between Chinese folk medicine and the folk medicines in other parts of the world.

While scientists, studying the anatomy and physiology of the human body, were developing the two great arts of acupuncture and moxibustion, herbalists were cataloguing plant-life into myriad combinations of remedies. As the two groups shared their knowledge, there emerged the basic principle of Chinese folk medicine: No two people are alike, and no single cure will work the same on everybody.

That's because no two people have the same *yin* and *yang*. In each person resides *yin,* the power of darkness (negative), and *yang,* the power of light (positive). Too much of either can result in illness. The object of Chinese herbal medicine is to bring each person's *yin* and *yang* into perfect harmony.

Chinese herbalism does not try to give each disease a label—names are used only for convenience. It is the patient's *yin* and *yang* that produce symptoms, and it is the individual symptoms that are treated, not the general disease.

Take the case of a simple cough. Western science prescribes the same remedies, regardless of the nature of the cough. Chinese medicine determines how the patient's *yin* and *yang* influence the cough, and then selects the proper herbal that will bring them into balance.

If the cough produces thick mucus, an herbal called *bakumonto* is prescribed. *Bakumonto* is a combination of six separate herbs. If the patient suffers from a dry cough, the medicine prescribed is *hangekobokuto,* which consists of five different herbs.

Does this mean, if you have a cough that produces thick mucus, you should run out to the nearest Oriental herb dispensary and buy a bottle of *bakumonto?* Hardly. Because only a trained herbalist can determine the precise nature of your particular *yin* and *yang,* and he alone can figure out the precise proportions that go into the formula.

This example of Oriental herbal medicine is one of many that fill volumes. They were built up over the centuries. That is not to say that only a trained herbalist can suggest the foods to take. Chinese folk medicine is also *preventive* medicine, and, to some extent, everyone can benefit from some of the herbs, regardless of the individual's *yin* and *yang*.

Hsun fu hua is the Chinese name for the herb elecampane, which grows in most parts of the world. Still widely used, elecampane is recommended as a promoter of strength, general tonic, carminative, diaphoretic, diuretic, antiseptic, and expectorant. The Chinese have taught the world that this herb makes an excellent remedy for chronic chest congestion, asthma, and bronchial coughs.

Dr. Lin first told me of its virtues, but he kept his word never to bore me with ingredients again. I had to find out for myself, many years later, that science is on the verge of extracting antibiotic elements from elecampane. Do you begin to see what Dr. Lin meant about sharing and learning from one another?

Another herb of many virtues is *huang lien*, the Chinese species of goldthread. Like its American relative, the Chinese variety takes its name from the gleaming tendrils of its root system. It is this delicate tangle of brilliant threads which furnishes the medicine that has been favored over the centuries for a variety of conditions.

Dr. Lin presented me with my first infusion of goldthread— four teaspoonfuls of the chopped, dried root in a quart of boiled water. After having been steeped for thirty minutes in a covered glass jar, the infusion was strained, cooled, and bottled. Best to keep refrigerated. Taken as directed, it is excellent for use in any of the following conditions:

Curative mouthwash: two tablespoons as a rinse and gargle after each meal and upon retiring. For the greatest effectiveness, keep in the mouth for about a minute and a half.

Diarrhea: a small wineglassful, sipped every three hours throughout the day and evening.

Swelling: small pads of cotton, soaked with the infusion and applied to the swollen parts.

Poor appetite: a jiggerful approximately half an hour before meals.

Also prominent in Dr. Lin's garden was the herb *ch'ang p'u,* known in America as sweet flag. After being picked, it is washed carefully and left in the sun until thoroughly dry. Then it's stored in the airiest, driest place in the household.

For a medicinal tea, sweet flag's dried, grated rhizome (underground stem) is placed in a preheated glass or china pot, and six ounces of boiling water are added. After it is steeped for five minutes, the tea is strained, and honey is added.

Sweet flag tea is recommended by the Chinese to stimulate the appetites of the elderly or to soothe colic in infants. It is also suggested as a remedy for sour stomach, indigestion, and heartburn, and as an aid in reducing inflammation of the gastric membrane.

Old-timers like Dr. Lin prefer the sweet flag remedy in its purest form. Simply cut off a small length of the dried rhizome, chew on it, and swallow the juice.

"To become a successful herbalist in China," Dr. Lin told me laughingly, during one of our numerous visits, "one must be an expert storyteller. Our herbal lore is steeped in legend—and who is to say where fact ends and fancy takes over?"

Like all civilizations, he went on, the Chinese have had their seekers of perpetual youth. Legends of success and failure abound, and out of some have emerged the mightiest of Chinese herb remedies.

One of Dr. Lin's favorite longevity stories tells of an ancient mandarin who was the image of youthfulness and vigor—at the age of one hundred and fifty! His twenty-four wives, plus an untold number of concubines, showered him with affection, making him the envy of all his male acquaintances. Everyone around him wondered about the secret of his superb youthfulness, but the mandarin would reveal nothing. When pressed beyond endurance, he would simply say, "I have two precious caskets."

Only after he died (at who knows what age?) was the mandarin's secret revealed. They were two famous herbs that, even today, are regarded in the Orient as youth elixirs. In one of the mandarin's caskets was *ginseng*, a plant with a history that reaches way back into antiquity. More than two thousand years ago, Confucius praised it as a curative and restorative. Princely sums are still being paid for it, and the wilder the species, the higher the price it commands.

Ginseng's American counterpart, the five fingers root, is a smaller plant but no lowlier than its Chinese cousin. The list of

ills that ginseng can remedy add up to a lengthy scroll. Emperor
Shen Nung, father of the first herbal, declared it "a tonic to the
five viscera, quieting the animal spirits, strengthening the soul,
allaying fear, expelling evil effluvia, brightening the eyes, opening the heart, benefiting the understanding, and, if taken for
some time, it will invigorate the body and prolong life."

In the second casket was *fo-ti-tieng*, less widespread than
ginseng today, but equally praised in Chinese herbal lore as a
rejuvenator of the glands and the brain cells. *Fo-ti-tieng* is also
known as *hydrocotyle Asiatica* and *gotu kola*. It is famed
throughout the Orient for its energizing effect on the brain. Two
fresh leaves a day are said to banish mental fatigue forever. It
also has wide use as a blood purifier and diuretic. The relentless
pain of rheumatism and neuritis give way to the eating of this
remarkable herb. (See next chapter.)

It was these two herbs that caused me to recall, many years
later, Dr. Lin's admonition that modern science has much to
learn from ancient herbalism—and vice versa. Each herb has
more than demonstrated its potential in the laboratory.

Like onion and garlic, ginseng gives off a radioactive aura
known as mitogenic radiations—similar to the radiations given
off by the human body. By replenishing the body's radiations,
ginseng apparently benefits and stimulates all the endocrine
glands, increasing their output of hormones. Mitogenic radiations also stimulate cell growth. Russian researchers have found,
in ginseng, elements that strengthen the heart and the nervous
system.

In *fo-ti-tieng*, according to French biochemist Jules Lepine,
exists "a rare tonic property which has a marked energizing effect on the nerves and brain cells." While performing research
financed by the French government, Professor Menier of the
Académie Scientifique discovered that *fo-ti-tieng* contains a vitamin that does not appear in any other herb. He named it vitamin X, the "youth vitamin."

While it is still in the early stages of scientific experimentation, much has been learned about its effects. In the tropics, it
has been effective against such diseases as leprosy and elephantia-
sis. A German scientist, Baron Gogern, found that only a few
leaves a day were needed to lessen the chances of nervous breakdown and to revitalize worn-out bodies and brains. Oil or juice

extracted from the plant reduces the fevers of bruises and swellings, including the rheumatic type.

Needless to say, the various uses of these herbs began centuries before the advent of modern science. But far and away, ginseng has been considered the most versatile.

As a heart strengthener, pulverized ginseng is blended with lard and dissolved in wine. For frailty in children, a dash of raw, minced ginseng is fed to them several times a day. A bowlful of its potion, mixed with honey, is said to stimulate blood circulation. An extract of ginseng mixed with an extract of celery root, is prescribed for stiff joints.

As you must have gathered by now, one needn't travel all the way to China to derive the benefits of her herbal remedies. Many a versatile Oriental plant, with its strange-sounding name, has its counterpart in Western kitchens or medicine cabinets.

Do you suffer from mild coughs? Heat or pain in the feet? Swellings or ulcers? You might try eating *t'ien men tung*, otherwise known as asparagus!

Many a victim of constipation, without realizing it, has relieved the condition with *ta huang*, one of the most ancient of Chinese remedies. It also goes by the same of rhubarb, which, in its medicinal form, has been used by Oriental herbalists to treat heart disease, dropsy, coughing or hoarseness, and numerous fevers.

Chiang—or ginger—is another heart strengthener. It is also recommended for nausea and dyspepsia.

An extract of *pi ma tze* has long been a favored Chinese laxative. In English, it is called the castor bean, from which the oil of the same is extracted. But the Chinese consider this bean far more versatile, as a cure for ulcers, swelling of the tongue, and certain forms of mild deafness. It has also been declared effective in the treatment of speech problems.

If you fancy foods sprinkled with cinnamon, you are already partaking of a Chinese remedy for excess gas, called *kuei*. Oriental herbalists also prescribe cinnamon to normalize the temperature of the liver and stomach.

Another remedy for excess gas is *jou tou k'ou*—the nutmeg. Chinese herbalists warn, however, that it should be avoided by pregnant women because it can cause miscarriage, and it should be eaten sparingly by everyone because it contains an oil that can produce poisons in the system.

Some Chinese food remedies are not quite so common outside her borders. In order to enjoy them, one must go to, of all places, a Chinese restaurant.

Soybean curds grace many a Chinese gourmet delight. Called *tou fu,* it is a Chinese remedy for jaundice. Ordinary soybeans, whose virtues I've extolled in my lectures and writings, go by the name of *ta tou.*

For certain cases of nausea, *chu hsun* is recommended. On Chinese menus, it is called bamboo sprouts and is served, roasted, with many meat dishes.

And who, once he's tasted it, can forget *li chih*—or litchi nuts —those delectable morsels served as after-meal snacks? In China, these fruits of the *li chih* herb are considered a great tonic.

Sha ch'i—shark's fins—are an ingredient of many dishes, especially soup. Chinese herbals describe them as a strength restorative. More esoteric, but equally tasty, is *yen wo,* or swallows' nests, a soup ingredient. It is used as a tonic for the sickly and the aged; this is not so wild an idea, since swallows build their nests of grasses and algae that contain many important vitamins. Chinese restaurants serve it as "bird's nest soup."

In certain provinces of China, farmers go out every morning to gather the leaves of a very special plant. Their legends say that this plant is most effective while still wet with the morning's dew and that it makes the best medicine when picked just after the first thunderstorm of the year. What is this plant called? *Tea!*

Yes, even tea *(ch'a)* has its place in the Chinese herbals. Cautioning that too much tea can cause sleeplessness, the ancients nevertheless ascribed many healing properties to tea leaves. When twisted into pill-shapes and boiled in onion water, they produce an infusion recommended for constipation. As a medicine, plain tea is prescribed for colds, headaches, dysentery, and weakened eyes.

Rice *(mi)*, the most basic of all Chinese foods, also has a place in herbal medicine. Remember, though, that the Chinese speak of rice in its brown, unpolished form only—not the empty-caloried, white version that's served in "civilized" lands. Steamed brown rice is said to benefit weakened sight and hearing and is also considered a thirst-quencher. And no wonder, since brown rice is rich in the B-complex vitamins.

In his basement, Dr. Lin had a unique laboratory. He spent hours on end there, extracting the essences of his garden herbs, grinding the roots into healing powders, creating tinctures from the leaves, flowers, and stems. It was also the place where he made copious notes of his analyses and comparisons with Western medicines, which he never rejected out of hand.

"Mark my word, Lelord," he said on more than one occasion. "The two disciplines will someday live side by side."

During a recent visit to China, I realized that his prophecy was on the verge of fulfillment. Modern Chinese medicine is indeed a blending of the old and the new. Throughout the Chinese countryside can be found a growing army of workers known as the "barefoot doctors." These men and women, untrained in the scientific disciplines, are students and practitioners of herbal healing. Their medicines come from plots where vast numbers of herbs are carefully cultivated.

There is no competition between the "barefoot doctors" and the formally trained physicians. The spirit is one of complete cooperation, with each group learning the best that the other has to offer.

In the medical detachments of most army regiments, vast numbers of herbs are grown both for treatment and education. Soldiers are taught to recognize them on sight and to convey their knowledge of them to the general population. In regimental hospitals, trained physicians work side by side with herbalists, comparing modern drugs with ancient herbs, combining them into the most effective medicines and preventives.

A typical dispensary in a Chinese hospital consists of herbal medicines—tinctures, powders, ampules, etc.—and modern antiseptics and antibiotics. Depending on the patient's condition, one or the other may be prescribed, or both together. Combinations of Chinese herbals and Western medications have been found particularly effective in the treatment of nephritis, ulcers, diabetes, and bronchial asthma. More illnesses are expected to be added to the list. The search for medicinal herbs has not ceased in China. Thousands of plants still lie undiscovered. Many, perhaps, deserve to remain undiscovered, but Chinese herbalism takes nothing for granted. Over the centuries, her practitioners have learned to leave no stone—or root—unturned in the quest for survival.

A SMATTERING OF CHINESE
HERBAL REMEDIES

**Coughs and
Chest Congestion**

Elecampane Cough Syrup

> 1 cup elecampane root
> 1 cup clover honey
> 1 cup water

Combine ingredients in a glass or enameled pan and bring to a quick boil. Reduce heat and simmer until root softens, then strain and bottle.

Dose: One tablespoon every four hours.

**Fever,
Dyspepsia,
Flatulence**

Sage Tea

> 1 ounce chopped sage leaves
> 2 ounces honey
> 3 tablespoons fresh lemon juice

Place all ingredients into a quart-size jar and fill to the top with boiling water. Cover and let stand for forty to fifty minutes. Strain through cheesecloth or muslin. Keep chilled. Pour over ice cubes for a cold drink, or reheat gently.

**Psoriasis,
Eczema,
Rheumatism,
Boils and Styes**

Burdock and Chamomile Decoction

> 1 ounce burdock seed, dried
> 1 ounce chamomile flowers, dried
> 1 pint water
> honey

Use a glass or enamel utensil. Simmer first two ingredients in boiling water for ten to fifteen minutes, covered. Strain through cheesecloth or muslin and sweeten to taste with honey. Store in refrigerator when cool.

Dose: Two ounces, four times daily for two weeks.

Digestion

ginseng powder
white of an egg

Use glass or enamel utensil. Blend ginseng powder with fresh egg white to make thick paste. Keep refrigerated.

Dose: One level teaspoonful three times a day.

21

The Secret of Prolonging Youth

No book on folk remedies could be considered complete without telling the rather strange story of a legendary plant considered by many to contain natural elements that may be of value in rewarding man's eternal struggle for prolongation of youth.

The plant in question undoubtedly contains organic minerals, vitamins, and auxins common to all green vegetation, but whether it contains some as-yet-undefined therapeutic element is open to speculation. Because of the almost tenacious belief in its properties which many have, it should be brought to the attention of the scientific world. But until scientific research confirms its values and either accepts or rejects the seemingly unfounded claims made for it, each reader must make his own decision!

Can emotion be explained—defined, analyzed, charted, its source pointed out with scientific accuracy? Hardly. But we experience unmistakable reactions to the mysterious force so named: We sense it, we feel it, we thrill to it—instinctively. Unerringly we know it when it stirs within us. We know that a mysterious, elusive urge is the cause, but we can put our finger *only* on the *effect*.

Just as elusive . . . just as mysterious . . . just as intriguing are travelers' tales of the effects of their *hydrocotyle Asiatica* herb on the natives of Ceylon. And while those primitive peoples know nothing of the whys and wherefores of the effect produced, they do claim that they seem *very real*.

After generations of experience, after ages of intimate, first-hand knowledge, many of the natives of the most vigorous Singhalese tribes are said to attribute their marvelous physique, their full vibrant physical existence, and their philosophical outlook on life partly to their precious *hydrocotyle Asiatica.*

And their sincere faith in this herb is fully reported by European and American travelers, explorers, scientists, and writers—some of whom have discovered native *hydrocotyle Asiatica* enthusiasts claiming to be over one hundred years of age who appear to be but sixty-five or seventy.

The nearest one can get to the answer is the possibility of a mysterious "something" which may reveal itself in the beneficial effects it has on the energy supply, the appetites, the emotions, and the general physical condition of humans and animals alike. Who knows but what that "something" may be a new vitamin source. Then, again, it may have an extraordinary mineral or unknown vital content; or it may be a combination of all! What that mysterious "something" is remains Nature's secret; so far, she has revealed it to no man.

Many newspaper and magazine articles have at various times written enthusiastically about the virtues of *hydrocotyle Asiatica,* basing their conclusions on the native stories and legends which it must be remembered are so far entirely without any recognized scientific substantiation. One of these writers, Vincent de Silva, writing about *hydrocotyle Asiatica* in the Ceylon *Daily News* said:

> Man's dream has always been to discover the secret of perpetual youth, and many men have devoted all their lives to this problem.
> We have heard of Ponce de Leon who sought restoration of youth from the waters of a charmed fountain in Florida; the Kintan of the Chinese; the Red Elixir of Geber, and the Vital Essence of Augsborg. More recently, a Swiss named Spalinger claimed to have found a serum which prolonged life to a hundred and fifty years.
> Instead of believing that the secret of perpetual youth could be thus obtained, they should have tracked an elephant in the wilds of Ceylon and observed what the behemoth ate for his lunch. Ten chances to one it would have been hydrocotyle asiatica. Had they done this, the world would be growing this life-giving plant as commonly as lettuce and there might not be on earth, today, any one with a body that could truthfully be termed senile.
> Hydrocotyle asiatica has a very ancient history. It was known to

writers of India and Ceylon hundreds of years ago—always as a longevity plant. It is a small herb that creeps along the ground, having fan-shaped leaves of a pale green color. It is claimed that this herb will increase the vitality of 70 and 80 to that of 40. The leaves have a marked energizing effect on the cells of the brain and can preserve it indefinitely.

Baron Gogern, the scientist, tells us that an old elephant, in captivity at Deshapur was once rejuvenated and bore a calf after hydrocotyle asiatica was sent for and mixed in her diet. A few of the leaves eaten every day will strengthen and re-vitalize wornout bodies and brains to a remarkable degree, preventing brain fag and nervous breakdown.

To realize the truth of these assertions, it is only necessary to look back a few hundred years into the medical history of the East.

If these reports were proved true they would astound all the civilized world. Whether they are true or without foundation, many will not wish to wait for proof and will want to experiment themselves with *hydrocotyle Asiatica* to personally determine its effect.

It is said that many a Singhalese almost worships *hydrocotyle Asiatica*. He swears by its beneficence, desiring it above many other foods to an almost fanatical degree. This extraordinary tribute to *hydrocotyle Asiatica* is corroborated by some European authorities who have known the facts for years.

It may seem to some a simple and easy matter to bring this herb from the jungle fastness on the other side of the world. Like other herbs, *hydrocotyle Asiatica* has its ripening and drying season, consequently any move to secure it in quantity must be made a long time in advance.

Gathering crews must be organized. They must be prepared to penetrate the jungle, to cut their way through the dense growth of the tropical forests, fighting the intense heat, torrential rainstorms, insects, wild beasts, and poisonous reptiles. Food, camp, working, and living equipment must be taken into the jungle, for the camp must remain long enough to sun-dry the herb on the ground.

Because of the difficulty in importing *hydrocotyle Asiatica,* the person who has an opportunity to procure a supply of this herb should consider himself fortunate.

What is there about this herb that inspires such strange tales from the Ceylonese natives? What precious gift has Nature locked within *hydrocotyle Asiatica,* if it really does any of the things the natives claim for it?

Nature has taught us to outfly the bird, outswim the fish, and outrun the deer—shall we then doubt that in her resources she holds for our discovery the secret of perfect physical life that she has revealed to these? She has taught us to chain rivers, harness the lightnings, and make a whispering gallery of sea and air. Is it then too much to expect that someday she may reveal to us her formula for more abundant power and more perfect living?

Have we found it in *hydrocotyle Asiatica;* in this plant from the jungle? The testimony of beasts and birds, of the natives and wise men of Ceylon and India, and a host of lay people of Europe and America seem to indicate to a reasoning mind that possibly we have. While science so far has not said yes or no, many have wanted to make their own personal experiments immediately without relying on the Ceylonese legends.

How precious is life! Though today be twenty-four hours of misery, "hope springs eternal in the human breast" and we carry on, ever looking for a brighter tomorrow in which we shall enjoy a fuller, richer physical existence. The virtues of *hydrocotyle Asiatica* have not yet been established, but we hope that someday science will turn its attention to this amazingly fabulous legendary herb.

For those fortunate enough to obtain the herb—a brighter tomorrow may lie in *hydrocotyle Asiatica.* As it is reported that countless Ceylonese natives seem to have found brighter days in the indefinable "something" which their systems may have drawn from *hydrocotyle Asiatica.* The reports from Ceylon indicate that the outward manifestations are evidenced by a general enhancement of the physical life; a brighter, keener mental activity; a restimulated ambition and a renewed optimistic outlook. Although it must be remembered that these reports are based entirely on folklore and hearsay.

Those who are below par physically and mentally—and who have the opportunity to experiment with *hydrocotyle Asiatica* may be able to tell whether they have experienced any of the following reactions reported in these words of a traveler in describing natives of Ceylon to whom this plant is available:

"I wish you could see these wonderful people, with their erect posture, their sharp eyes and velvety skin. Their limbs are as if carved from ebony, of splendid proportion, their chests deep, their bodies firm, with gracefully curved hips and flat abdomens. The rhythm of their motions, their gracefulness and poise, their stately bearing, the intelligence of their eyes and their pleasing laughter all show them blessed with an extraordinary physique."

To quote again from Vincent de Silva's article:

> It is the belief of the Singhalese and the Indians also, that only a few leaves of this herb are necessary, daily, to bring about a gradual return to health and strength, provided the body is exposed to the sun. If this is eaten daily, it is said, disorders like rheumatism, neuritis and nervous breakdown can be banished entirely from the constitution. It is claimed that hydrocotyle asiatica will increase the span of life by many years, developing a brain incapable of breaking down for a very long time.

To many, the above will seem "too good to be true," and it must be emphasized that so far there has been no evidence from any recognized scientific source confirming (or denying) the Ceylonese reports, perhaps because the reports have not been sufficiently established to warrant scientific investigation.

On the other hand, hundreds are becoming interested enough to make a personal experiment with *hydrocotyle Asiatica,* and undoubtedly many more will be pleased to know that this herb is available in tablet form for experimental use.

Epilogue

Give Nature a Chance
(THE NEED FOR PREVENTIVE REMEDIES)

For nearly a half century I have been collecting and evaluating the preventive and curative home remedies and natural food supplements used by man in his fight for better health.

In the beginning, the search involved no more travel than the short distance to Grandma's herb and flower garden where it all began when I was a boy.

As an adult, my work in nutrition became worldwide. Visits to Europe and Australia have become routine, with occasional journeys to Russia, China, Japan, Africa, and other countries. Whenever my busy schedule of lecturing permitted, I left the cities and made side trips to isolated villages where I talked to the old-timers about the food they ate to keep them healthy and asked about their native folk remedies.

These spare-time excursions changed to a full-scale intensive search when my editor asked me to write a book on international folk medicine . . . the book you now hold.

The remedies in Grandma's notebooks, and those in my own collection, were enough to form the nucleus of several chapters. With so much work already done, I thought in those first days of enthusiasm that the rest of the book would practically write itself.

Had I turned down a page in my memory, I would have been reminded that no book of mine has *ever* "practically written itself"! Or even come close to it. All of them have taken long, exhausting months—sometimes years—of study, research, and experimentation before the actual writing ever began. In looking over the material I had, and adapting some of the older remedies to modern use, I realized that many more would be needed if I was to write this book as I began to visualize it.

There were still some countries left on my must-see list, and I knew that I wouldn't be satisfied until I visited them. I was particularly eager to visit the areas that had no doctors and to find out what home treatments were used, how well they worked, and which ones could be adapted to our needs.

Often a trip to some remote area did not result in my finding a usable remedy. But when even one safe, economical, and effective remedy was found, it made up for all the wasted trips.

Medical care on a mass basis has become a manifold problem that involves the already prohibitive and still soaring cost of hospital care, the continuing increase in doctors' fees, the scarcity of doctors in many rural areas as acute as that in some of the underdeveloped countries I visited, and the overspecialization of those in the cities.

The overspecialization problem recently hit a friend of mine in a very tender spot—his pocketbook! When he went to his personal physician with four separate complaints, none of them major, he was treated in the doctor's office for one, given two prescriptions for high-priced drugs, and referred to three different specialists for the other disorders.

"I ended up wasting a lot of time waiting for appointments," he told me, "and paying four doctor bills instead of one. And those expensive specialists didn't do a damn thing for me that our old family doctor couldn't have done in one visit! In addition, the recommended total of nine prescription drugs cost sixty-two dollars."

Dr. Leslie T. Webster, chairman of the pharmacology department at Northwestern University Medical School, believes that we have become a drug-oriented society, and in his opinion both doctor and patient are to blame. "The average physician writes prescriptions for seventy-five percent of his patients," he says, "and too many are for drugs that are unnecessary, ineffective as recommended, and sometimes downright dangerous."

The danger grows as, each year, more and stronger drugs come on the market.

Haphazard self-medication with drugs is not the answer. But a knowledge of preventive remedies and the use of safe, natural home medication can help prevent and correct many minor disorders. An increasing number of doctors are beginning to recognize this fact, and some of them are speaking out on the subject. One of them is Dr. Daniel Freedman, chairman of the psychiatry department at the University of Chicago, who says, "Societies have to self-medicate themselves. If we didn't, we'd have to go to a specially trained person for everything."

Dr. Robert D. Conn, chairman of the department of medicine at Southern Illinois University, has stated, "The public has grown to expect the doctor to be responsible for them when they should be responsible for themselves. Science can determine what good health is and develop a mechanism for achieving it, but the responsibility is the patients'. It's up to them, not the doctor, to take corrective action and get themselves back in shape."

However, a word of common sense is in order: It would be foolhardy to expect folk remedies and home preventive measures to be the answer to all of our ills. They aren't, and no such claims are made for them. In earlier chapters I emphasized the need for professional diagnosis and treatment in conditions that require it, and that need should not be ignored.

But for conditions that lend themselves to home treatment, why not start with one or two remedies that meet your requirements and give them a fair trial? When you're satisfied that they work, you'll want to add others to the list. But remember that natural remedies work more slowly than drugs, so give them a little time and don't get discouraged if you can't see *immediate* results.

A concept once taught in medical school is that of "dynamic equilibrium." Maybe it's still taught and we just don't hear about it anymore, though it's just as valid today as it ever was. The processes of the body are never at rest. In spite of the obstacle courses we make them run, the odds often stacked against them by the changes they're subjected to in both the external and internal environment, they never figuratively throw in the towel and say, "I give up!" Instinctively they roll with the punches, constantly changing and striving to keep us well by maintaining a general equilibrium.

Why not give your dynamic equilibrium a chance to keep you well by supplying it with a wholesome, balanced diet and the added benefits of nature's healing remedies?

General Index

Recipe Index